CANCER CURE

via DNA

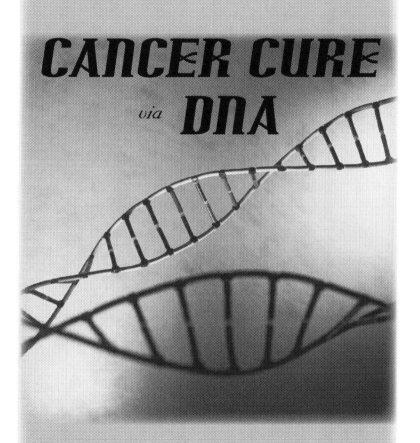

ANTHONY J LUKSAS PHD

iUniverse, Inc.
Bloomington

Cancer Cure via DNA

The information, ideas, and suggestions in this book are not intended as a substitute for professional medical advice. Before following any suggestions contained in this book, you should consult your personal physician. Neither the author nor the publisher shall be liable or responsible for any loss or damage allegedly arising as a consequence of your use or application of any information or suggestions in this book.

iUniverse books may be ordered through booksellers or by contacting:

iUniverse
1663 Liberty Drive
Bloomington, IN 47403
www.iuniverse.com
1-800-Authors (1-800-288-4677)

Because of the dynamic nature of the Internet, any web addresses or links contained in this book may have changed since publication and may no longer be valid. The views expressed in this work are solely those of the author and do not necessarily reflect the views of the publisher, and the publisher hereby disclaims any responsibility for them.

Any people depicted in stock imagery provided by Thinkstock are models, and such images are being used for illustrative purposes only.

Certain stock imagery © Thinkstock.

ISBN: 978-1-4759-6802-6 (sc)
ISBN: 978-1-4759-6801-9 (hc)
ISBN: 978-1-4759-6800-2 (e)

Library of Congress Control Number: 2012923762

Printed in the United States of America

iUniverse rev. date: 1/29/2013

This Book is dedicated to my wife Gerrie for putting up with me for 4 years during the writing of this Book. Also, to David Hill for the suggestion and encouragement to write this Book.

TABLE OF CONTENTS

INTRODUCTION

SINCE THE DAY IN 1959 when I took my first course in Microbiology, I became intrigued by the intricacies and control of DNA. In 1953, Watson and Crick discovered the alpha helix of the DNA molecule. In the 1960's DNA became the seat of inheritance. . Everything one is, is in the DNA. The only question obviously is the soul that makes us different from the rest of living things on this planet. It is the belief of believers that the soul is implanted at the time of conception. Saying that there is no soul or that is done later is just begging the question. Even now, nonbelievers have to admit that humans have abilities that no animal on this planet possess and, as late as 2006, Francis S. Collins, in his book, "The Language of God", admits after identifying the genetic code of man, that what and how the soul which is external from DNA comes and makes man different from the other mammals on this planet.

In my first course, I learned how DNA is transmitted between microbes by such processes as Transduction and Recombination. These processes and others confer on the microbe new capabilities that the microbe did not have before.

In subsequent courses I learned the viral transmission of new genetic material into a colony of bacteria. Essentially, the viruses [in bacteria they are called bacteriophages] infecting a bacterial colony will destroy most of the bacteria, but approximately every 1,000,000, the virus remains in the bacteria. The bacteriophage in the bacteria can stay in the cytoplasm as an extrachromosomal element called plasmid, or be integrated into the bacterial DNA as an episome. The bacteriophage can express itself or lay dormant. Under the right conditions, the virus as a plasmid or as episome can express itself. The expression is either good or bad for the bacteria. It can provide survival mechanism to the bacteria or it can express itself and destroy the bacteria by taking over the DNA of the bacteria and reproducing into many bacteriophages.

In humans, we acquire genetic material mostly via viral infections that may be beneficial to vital to cope with the dangerous environment, or bad by destroying the cell and also in some cases the surrounding cells.

The acquisition of new genetic material takes place by infection with viruses or for that matter, bacteria. As in bacteria, so it is in humans, every 1,000,000 cells that a virus destroys, one survives and the virus becomes part of the cell. This viral acquisition and integration into the human DNA can be transmitted through generations in the sperm DNA or the egg DNA, or acquired during infection.

The acquired DNA may remain in the cell for generations, or be expressed by subjecting the cell to inducing chemicals and subsequently to promoting chemicals. In many cases, but not all, the viral infection once expressed can destroy the cell or cause the cell to escape the control of the body, and the cell multiplies as either benign or a cancerous tumor. The body's defense usually identifies that cell or that growth as non-self and destroys the cell or the colony. Tumors that have a "cloaking" mechanism that prevents the bodies defense systems from identifying the growth, and if cancerous, destroy the individual if no intervention.

Chemotherapy and Radiation delay the inevitable since these processes destroy most of the cancerous cells, but not all. If the cancer has metastasized, radiation only destroys the target cancer growth, and not all cells of the cancer. Chemotherapy should also destroy the metastasized cells/growth but again, not all.

In addition, in destroying the cancer cells, chemotherapy and radiation also destroys the immune system, and since these chemicals can be also by themselves carcinogenic, can cause other cancers. At times, cancer can reverse and disappear after chemotherapy or radiation or both. It has been attributed to divine intervention. It is routine to say that God, through divine intervention does perform miracles, but there may be other explanations. Divine intervention is there and can take place especially if one is a believer. Therefore, due to ones belief in divine intervention, the immune system recognizes the cancer as non-self and destroys it. It also may be that chemotherapy and radiation in the process of destroying the cancer cell "unlocks" the very nature of why the immune system did not recognize the cancer cell. Now, once recognized, as non-self starts to destroy the cancer.

It is very important to note that cancers form in individuals throughout one's lifetime, but the body recognizes the cells as non-self and destroys the cells. There are many diseases where the immune system starts to destroy so called healthy cells, like Rheumatoid Arthritis, Rheumatic Fever, and Lupus. We will touch on this area in the following pages.

In the situations where the body does not recognize the cancer cells as non self and allow these cells to grow into cancer and destroy the individual, there are ways of causing recognition as non self more directly than by chemotherapy, radiation or divine intervention.

Remembering Pasteur and his work with T.B. and Rabies and combining the recently [in the last 40 years] introduced Genetic Engineering. I believe there are ways of causing the bodies defenses to recognize and destroy the cancer. It is all to do with removing the "cloaking" mechanism from the cancer cell. You will have to read the following pages of this book to get the gist of how to do it.

CHAPTER 1
DNA, RNA AND PROTEIN

IT IS ESSENTIAL TO understand DNA, RNA and Proteins to proceed in understanding of the contents of this book. DNA is the seat of inheritance of all that we are minus the soul. One cannot explain the soul by DNA. Also, as we get into the details of DNA, RNA and Proteins, we determine the results that they produce, but there is no explainable reason why these organic molecules do what they do. That is to say, once the different atoms of carbon, oxygen, hydrogen, phosphorus and nitrogen are put together into monomers, then these monomers into polymers to make DNA, RNA and Protein (proteins contain in addition sulfur as part of some amino acids the building blocks of protein).

The laws of nature dictate the DNA, RNA and Proteins will function without exception in performing the function that was intended. Do not ask why and how, only that they do what they do. It is also interesting to know that carbon plays a major role in biochemistry that includes DNA, RNA and Proteins. Carbon is the backbone and the predominant atom in all of biochemistry – the study of molecules that are found in living systems on earth. How these molecules are made in the cell

Anthony J Luksas PhD

be it bacterial or human is the study of biochemistry and cell physiology and related courses, and will not be discussed in this book. We will proceed from the point where these molecules have been produced.

There are only 20 different amino acids, figure 1 and 2, therefore many of the triplets code for some of the amino acids more than once. There are three triplets that do not code for amino acids, but are used to terminate a polypeptide chain.

FIGURE 1

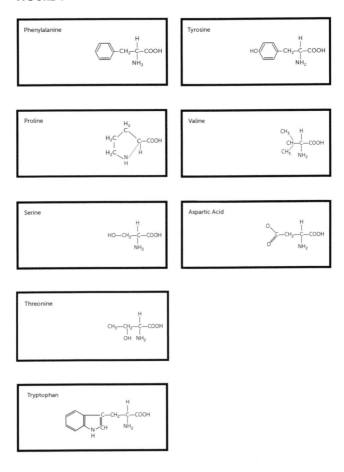

FIGURE 2

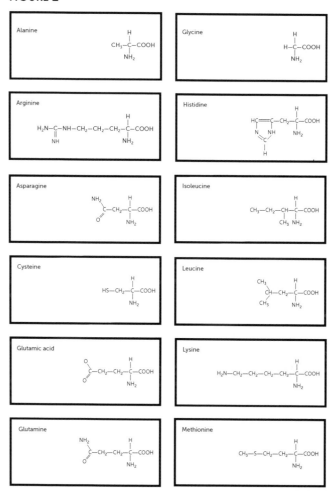

All DNA in all species on this earth consist of the 4 mononucleotides. The ration of each varies in species, but only these nucleotides are present.

Deoxyribonuleic acid (DNA) contains 2 purine bases – adenine (A), guanidine (G) and 2 pyrimidine bases – thyamine (T) and cytosine (C). Ribonuclaic acid [RNA] contains 2 purine bases

– adenine [A] and guanidine [G], and 2 pyrimidine bases – cytosine [C] and uridine [U], Figure 3.

FIGURE 3

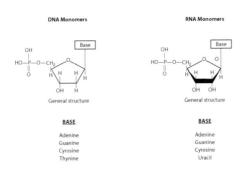

The bases are attached to the No. 1 carbon of deoxyribose, the phosphoric acid is attached to the No. 5 carbon.

When the DNA polymer is formed the phosphoric acid is chemically bonded to the No. 3 carbon of the next mononucleotide (composed of nitrogenous base, five carbon sugar and phosphoric acid), and so forth. Now, if a gene (definition of a gene: segment of DNA that directs the production of a complete protein) directs the production of a complete protein of 100 amino acids, that gene is composed of at least 300 nucleotides. It has been determined experimentally that it takes 3 nucleotides to determine an amino acid. Therefore, 4 to the 3power = 64, and theoretically can determine 64 different amino acids, Figure 4.

FIGURE 4

	A	C	G	U
A	UAU Tyr UAC Tyr	UCU Ser UCC Ser	UGU Cys UGG Cys	UUU Phe UUC Phe
	UAA UAG	UCA Ser UCG Ser	UGA UGG Trp	UUA Leu UUG Leu
C	CAU His CAC His	CCU Pro CCC Pro	CGU Arg CGC Arg	CUU Leu CUC Leu
	CAA Gln CAG Gln	CCA Pro CCG Pro	CGA Arg CGG Arg	CUA Leu CUG Leu
G	AAU Asn AAC Asn	ACU Thr ACC Thr	AGU Ser AGC Ser	AUU Ile AUC Ile
	AAA Lys AAG Lys	AGA Thr ACG Thr	AGA Arg AGG Arg	AUA Ile AUG Met
U	GAU Asp GAC Asp	CCU Ala CCC Ala	GGU Gly GGC Gly	GUU Val GUC Val
	GAA Asp GAG Glu	CCA Ala GCG Ala	GGA Gly GGG Gly	GUA Val GUG Val

Microorganisms that do not separate the DNA from cytoplasm by a membrane are called prokaryotes (prokaryotes are bacteria). In prokaryotic cells like bacteria, the DNA is a single chromosome exceeding 2×10 to the ninth in molecular weight. That chromosome is composed of 5-6 million nucleotides and, if 3 nucleotides determine an amino acid, therefore there are 3 million triplets, and if 100 amino acids compose a complete protein, therefore one gene approximately. There are, in single bacteria, approximately 30,000 genes. A virus as a comparison has approximately up to 200 genes depending on the virus; as we said above, in prokaryotic cells there is an apparent division between the cell components and the chromosomes. There is an attachment of the DNA on the chromosome in the inside of the prokaryotic cell membranes, but no separation by a membrane of DNA from cytoplasm. Eukaryotic cells contain, depending on the species, several to many chromosomes. The chromosomes consist of two double stranded DNA molecules. The DNA in eukaryotic cells is very complex and packed into chromosomes. The eukaryotic germ cells consist of one double stranded DNA.

In eukaryotic cells, there is a clear division between the chromosomes and the rest of cell components. The chromosomes are in an area separated by a membrane and that is called the nucleus. The rest of the cell area is called the cytoplasm.

Mitochondria have its own DNA. It is the cell's energy mill. It is the current belief that there existed a symbiotic relationship between prokaryotes and eukaryotes, until the prokaryote became part of the eukaryote as mitochondria. Mitochondrial DNA is single stranded like bacteria, and it divides like bacteria. The same appears to be also with chloroplasts of plants.

Ribonucleic acid (RNA) is composed of adenine (A), granine (G), cytosine (C) and uracil (U) bases, each attached to ribose, also attached to ribose are phosphoric acid. Poly RNA is created by one ribose unit with attached base at position one on the ribose and phosphoric acid attached at position five which reacts with another ribose on position three and so forth. During the process of transcription, DNA makes RNA. After transcription – messenger RNA (mRNA), as this RNA is known. There are other types of RNA made by DNA also, but mRNA is needed to translate (or make) protein. The other RNA's are ribosomal RNA (gamma RNA) and transfer RNA (t RNA).

During the process of transcription, DNA makes RNA. After transcription mRNA attaches to a ribosome in the cytoplasma, and is used to make protein.

In 1953, Watson and Crick deduced the double helical structure of DNA. The dogma that evolved from that and other developments after were the following:

1. Replication – the coupling of DNA to form identical DNA molecules

2. Transcription – the process by which DNA is transcribed (made) into RNA. The RNA then attaches to ribosome.
3. Translation – the process by which genetic message is decoded and converted into the 20-letter alphabet of protein structure.

To go into details as to the "process" of replication, transcription and translation is a mute point. There are many advanced courses given at the universities, but that knowledge is not essential to the understanding of this book.

The knowledge of how each process works, and the processes of making and transporting these molecules are unknown – it just happens. We know that these processes take place by looking at the results. Why do these formed molecules do what they do, and how do they do what they do is a mystery. Some people of higher learning try to explain not why but how by using thermodynamics and organic and inorganic chemistry of simple molecules, but in my opinion, to no avail.

Next area of understanding that will help to follow the developments in this book is what is the structure of proteins, composition of proteins, how they are made and what is their function. First, RNA makes essentially all proteins. There are some proteins that will be discussed later that are made directly by DNA – repressor proteins; but RNA makes the various proteins in the cell other than repressor proteins.

Proteins are composed of amino acids that are made by enzymes, which are proteins. Some enzymes require other molecules or elements to function. There are 20 different amino acids, as figure 1 and 2 indicates.. Amino acids can be described as a carbon atom to which are attached a hydrogen, amine (NH2), carboxyl (COOH) and an R group. The R group is what makes the amino acids different from each other. There are 20 amino acids; all proteins consist of these 20 amino acids. There are 15 neutral amino acids, 2 acidic amino acids and 3 basic amino acids. Some of these amino acids may be modified by enzymatic action like prolein into hydroxi prolein. If this modification was not made or partially made, collagen would not have a three dimensional structure, and would not function as the glue of biological systems, The blood vessels would start bleeding, organs would start to fall apart. This process is known as Scurvy. At a certain point in this process, the biological unit like man would die.

Good collagen is made by hydroxilation of proline. The enzyme (protein) requires vitamin C to function; since without vitamin C, the enzyme does not function. Many enzymes require co-factors. These co-factors are the various vitamins and some elements. Amino acids are made into proteins by the carboxyl group of one amino acid reacting with amine group of another amino acid and so forth. The bond formed between two amino acids is called a peptide bond.

Once a specific mRNA is produced from a DNA gene, it travels to a ribosome where it is translated into protein. How long the protein chain is, composition of amino acids, and position of these amino acids within the protein chain determines the function of the protein chain. As an example of the specificity of amino acids and the position of that amino acid is sickle cell anemia. Sickle cell hemoglobin is different from normal hemoglobin by only one amino acid. Hemoglobin has an alpha chain and a beta chain. The alpha chain, no change, but in the beta chain at position six-glutamine acid is replaced by valine. There are many examples.

It is interesting to note that the following is an additional piece of info to strongly suspect that mitochondrial is of bacterial origin. The mitochondria produces its own RNA and ribosomes and the synthesis of protein is characteristically like the protein synthesis apparatus similar to bacteria. This and the DNA of mitochondria strongly support the hypothesis that mitochondria are from symbiotic or parasitic bacteria resulting during evolution of eukaryotic cells.

Proteins that are produced by different RNA's on ribosomes, become enzymes, structural protein, immune protein etc. These proteins produce all the components of the cell by producing the various biochemical – lipids, lipoproteins, vitamins, carbohydrates etc.

CHAPTER 2
BACTERIAL, PLANT, ANIMAL
AND HUMAN VIRUSES

THROUGHOUT THE FOLLOWING CHAPTERS we will explore the DNA and RNA viruses as the cause of Cancer. Bacteria do not develop so called "Cancers", but the results that bacteriophages (bacterial viruses) impart to the bacteria can be considered as Cancer. The bacteriophages confer on the bacteria that allow them to either survive in inanimate environment or living environment by producing toxins that causes the living environment to die and degrade into components that the bacteria can live on.

Therefore, bacterial plasmids and bacteriophages play a key role in the bacteria as causing either pathogenicity, or, toxin production that allows the bacteria to survive in a hostile living environment.

In cases studied, pathogens or toxin producing microbes were shown to possess a large segment of DNA – (35-170) kilobases. This includes a number of virulent genes that are not present in non-pathogens.

In enteropathogenic E.coli, there is extra DNA. How is this determined? The DNA is analyzed by hydrolyzing to gene level the DNA, and subjecting the genes to electrophoreses, not unlike DNA analysis in forensics.

In the enteropathogenic E.coli there are extra genes that do not exist in regular E.coli. Up to 10% of the bacteria in the human intestinal track are regular E.coli. Similar possibilities exist in Shigella, tetanus , B.anthraces, C.diptheria, S. pyrogenes, C.botulinum, enterohemorehagic E.coli and many others. The bacteria have to acquire a specific gene or genes to become pathogenic.

Also, extra chromosomal genes encoding other virulence factors are common among gram-negative pathogens ranging from plant pathogens to human like human Helicobacter pylori. Therefore, pathogenicity is due to acquisition of plasmids, lysogenic phages and transposons; and not to some form of adoption by the pathogens.

The following scale depicts viral infections:

Pathogens	HIV	Cancer	Degenerative Diseases
Instant effect and fast growth	and related viruses	may take 20-30 years to develop can be fast growth after that or slow growth	May take sometime or years to have an effect on nerve cells, muscle cells etc.

Depending on the plasmid or bacteriophage in bacterial situation, the end result is better for the bacteria, and can be bad for higher organisms like plants, animals and man, but in human cells when viral infections take place and most of the cells infected are destroyed, but, some survived by the virus becoming a prophage. Since plants, animals and man genetically are very complicated, and if interactions do take place in higher organisms it is similar to bacterial infections with bacteriophages, then there are interactions that we do not know anything about, until or unless they manifest themselves in a form of a disease, and we have the capacity to identify it as a disease.

Not much is known about the cancers in plants. The crown gall tumor is caused by Agrobacterium tumefaciens. This organism is closely related to Rhizobium which depending on species fixes nitrogen in symbiotic association with leguminous plants. The leguminous plants that fix nitrogen when in symbiotic association with Rhizobium are alfalfa, clover, peas, beans, peanuts, soybeans and vetch. The association forms nodules on the roots of the plant. The bacteria and the plants can grow separately, but the bacteria will disappear from the soil if no leguminous plants are growing for a long time. The bacteria fix nitrogen only in association with the plant. There does not appear to be any genetic material transferred from the bacteria to the plant or from plant to bacteria.

It is intracellular symbionts that infects root cells that are tetraploid (cells that have four sets of chromosomes), normal diploid cells are usually destroyed by the infection. The single cell swells and the bacteria multiply and form the root modules.

If a species of Rhizobium cannot infect or if infected cell does not fix nitrogen, then by transferring the DNA from infection and nitrogen fixing by DNA mediated transformation, the non infected or non nitrogen fixing species can become infective and nitrogen fixing. Rhizobium is also attacked by bacteriophages that lyse the cells.

It is possible, but at this writing not known, if Rhizobium lysogenic state exist and that if the proper phage infects and creates the lysogenic state that is the state of the Rhizobium [in a lysogenic state] fixes nitrogen.

Agrobacterium tumefaciens causes a tumor like growth in plants called crown gall tumor. In this situation only the crown gall tumor starts, destroying the bacteria does not stop the development of the tumor. Recent experiments strongly suggest that the bacterial DNA becomes associated or integrated into the DNA of the plant cell that causes the tumor. A plasmid called Ti (tumor-inducing) is transferred from the Agrobacterium tumefaciens to the plant cell. It is then stable in the tumor tissue. It has been also shown that all oncogenic strains of Agrobacterium contain Ti plasmid. If the strains containing Ti plasma are cured of Ti plasmid, the cured strains do not induce tumors. But, if the Ti Plasmid is reintroduced into the bacteria by DNA transformation or conjugation, the resulting strain infects, transfers the Ti plasmid to plant cells and tumor develops. This is basic knowledge found in any microbiology book.

Viruses are known to induce tumors in animals. It has been determined that in fowl, sarcomas and avian leucosis are caused by infecting viruses. Rabbit papillomas is also caused by viruses. Two different leukemia's in mice are caused by viruses. All of these cancers can be induced by filterable agents. Investigation by Raus of sarcoma in fowl, and that disease bares his name – Raus sarcoma.

Here also there is absorption and penetration of the cell not unlike in bacteria. There are receptor sites for viruses that infect mammalian cells. Little is known about the molecular reaction in the absorption process.

Following absorption, a series of events occur which includes penetration and uncoating of the virus. This results in liberation into the host cytoplasm of viral DNA.

The host enzymes, ribosomes and host DNA are utilized in transcription and translation of viral DNA into viral RNA. Some viruses DNA have DNA dependent RNA polymerase.

The mechanism of viral DNA and RNA replication is as described for the bacterial bacteriophages. Many animal viruses can infect animal cells, and more than one type of virus can infect the same animal cell. When the cell either releases the complete virus by budding or by lysis, the resulting viruses can have DNA from both viruses; this is called Recombination. Recombination has been shown to occur in several groups of DNA viruses. Recombination has also been recorded in two RNA viruses – influenza (myxovirus) and polio (picarno virus).

Two types of viral release mechanisms are found in mammalian cell.

1. Release by envelop derived from the mammalian cell membrane, but prior to extrusion, a number of viral protein are incorporated into the cell membrane. The envelope contains both viral and host material. All lipids are derived from the host membrane.
2. Other viruses are released by ruptures in the membrane of the cell and the cell dies. In No. 1 above, the "budding off" takes place, and the cell may continue to multiply during the process and survive indefinitely – knows as "steady-state infection". Clones of cells may develop that multiply and release viruses by "budding off".

It is possible therefore, that in metastasis that not cells is released or breaks off and travels via blood or lymphatic route to other parts of the body, but it could be that

#1 or #2 above take place and reinfect and develop cancer at distal parts of the body.

The growth of animal tissue is regulated with limited growth. In a rare event, a cell escapes regulation and multiplies unrestrained and develops into a mass. These masses are called tumors or neoplasms. The development of tumors is called neoplasia.

Some tumors, like papilloma's (warts) are benign. Other tumors are malignant; destroy the cells or organ where the malignancy develops. Malignant tumors send cells or viruses to distal parts of the body to form other more malignant tumors. Cancer is malignant tumor. There are variety of cancers, and they are in the majority by adding a named suffix – oma to the name of the tissue the tumor is associated with lymphoma – cancer of lymphoid tissue, sarcoma – cancer of fleshy non epithelial tissue, adenocarcinoma is a cancer of glandular tissue. Exception: leukemia is the cancer of the white blood cells.

Both RNA and DNA viruses can induce tumors. The RNA viruses include the mouse leukemia's, Raus sarcoma virus, and mouse mammary tumor viruses. The DNA viruses include Shope Papilloma virus and the Polyoma virus.

One of these viruses SV-40 (simian virus 40) was discovered as a contaminant in monkey kidney-cell cultures – used to produce polio vaccine. Transformation of normal cells into tumor cells can be demonstrated in tissue cultures. If a suspension of tumor virus particles is used to infect a susceptible tissue culture, some or most of the cells exhibit unregulated growth. Normal cells in tissue culture when growing and come in contact with another cell or cells, they stop dividing. That phenomenon is known as contact inhibition, and eventually form a monolayer of cells. But, if cells exhibit unregulated growth, they will continue growing and if the transformed cells are introduced into a body they will initiate tumors.

The efficiency of transformation varies among tumor viruses. Raus sarcoma virus transforms almost all cells in tissue culture, while other tumor viruses may only transform one cell in a million cells.

Transformed cell can be shown to contain the virus even though in viral induced tumor or in tissue culture no detectable viral particles are found. If transformed cells are grown with susceptible cells under conditions that promote fusion, the normal cells may become infected and liberate viral particles. Therefore, under these conditions a complete viral genome is expressed.

Raus sarcoma virus will transform both chicken and mammalian cells in tissue culture. Transformed chicken cells continue to produce active virus, but the mammalian cells do not. If mammalian cells are injected into chicks, the chicken tumors are formed and these produce active virus particles. In polyoma virus and other tumor viruses, the above results are the same. Presence of viruses can be demonstrated by cell fusion. Some transformed cells shed viruses and others do not.

The analogy of transformation of bacteria by bacteriophages and transformation by DNA of mammalian tissue by viruses is similar. The following changes are evident in both 1. Many of the viral genes are repressed or are not expressed. 2. Immunity to infection with similar virus. 3. The physiology of the host cell is altered, since some of the viral genes are expressed. The lysogenized bacteria and transformed animal cells often show changed cell surface properties and the animal cells lose contact inhibition. The loss of contact inhibition may be the direct cause or indirect in initiating neoplasia. It is highly likely that cancers are caused by viruses. There are viruses that a body inherits in its DNA from birth or are acquired after birth during viral infections.

Why in some people these viruses cause cancer and in others they do not is still a mystery. Obviously, many theories are proposed, like carcinogen theory that somehow causes the virus to become active and produce cancers. For example, cigarette smoke produces many carcinogens that should cause cancer, and in some individuals it does, but not all.

CHAPTER 3
BACTERIOPHAGES, BACTERIAL
PROPHAGES AND LYSOGENY

IN THIS CHAPTER THE interaction of bacterial viruses and bacteria is explored, and the possibility that similar type of interactions take place in vertebrates and man, but probably more complex. The exploration is not in depth, but only examples were chosen to indicate that even at the level of bacteria DNA and RNA activity is very complex. It is not necessary to understand but only to appreciate the complexity that DNA and RNA are capable of. Even people that work in this area do not understand what is happening and how.

In the previous chapter, we discussed the seat of inheritance or DNA. We also looked at how the information from DNA is made into RNA. RNA migrates to the ribosomes where it makes protein. There is a lot more to the discussion of DNA, much more details are known, as a matter of fact, books have been written but, for our needs of understanding, the info in the previous chapter should suffice in understanding of what follows.

Now, what is known about the interaction of viruses with living organisms is derived from viruses interacting with bacteria. These viruses are called bacteriophages.

It is interesting to note the respective size of what we are dealing with.

The respective size of human cells, bacterial cells, and viruses is as follows; To give you first how these cells and viruses are measured, we need to review the classifications of measurement. One meter is approximately one yard; one millimeter is 1/1000 of a meter. One micron is 1/1000 of a millimeter. A nanometer or mill micron is one thousandth of a micron, and one nanometer is 10 Å. Now, a liver cell is approximately 200,000 Å. A bacterial cell like E. coli is 20,000 Å, and viruses are from 72 – 5000 Å.

How do we know that these cells and viruses exist? Liver cells and other cells are evaluated by a light microscope. Bacterial cells are also evaluated by light microscope at about 1000 X magnification. But to see bacterial cells you need to stain the cells. Yeast and molds can also be seen by light microscope. Molds normally with no staining since they are significantly larger than bacteria, yeast are best evaluated by staining. Yeast is intermediate in size between bacteria and molds.

Viruses can be seen only by electron microscopes. Some of the larger viruses, like tobacco mosaic virus, the outer coating can be seen by a good 1000 X light microscope.

Most of the developments and interactions of DNA had been derived from studying bacteria to bacteria interactions and viruses to bacteria interactions. We will not need to use visualization since the interactions are studied biochemically or more specifically by genetic engineering of DNA, RNA, and proteins. The size information is provided to give the reader an idea of relative size that we will be dealing with.

Now, Twort in England and d He Relle in France working independently demonstrated that filterable agents that pass through 0.1 µ filter (bacteria are removed or filtered out with 0.1 µ filter) could infect and destroy bacteria's. These filterable agents today are known as bacteriophages or phages. And because of the ease of growth of bacteria, phages can be cultured much more readily than many other viruses that infect animals or plants. This gave much knowledge and understanding of viruses. First, viruses are considered not alive, since they need a living-dividing cell to replicate. Virus particle [virion, phages] consists of a single type of nucleic acid (DNA or RNA, surrounded by protein codes [capsid]. In some cases also by an outer layer or envelope which contains carbohydrates and lipids.

In viruses, nucleic acid (DNA, RNA) may occur as double stranded DNA, single stranded DNA, double stranded RNA, or single stranded RNA. A single virion can direct the synthesis of dozens or even up to as many as thousands of similar viruses within a host cell.

The steps of replication are similar for all viruses that so far have been examined, same applies to bacteria, yeast, molds, algae, plants and animals cells.

A viral DNA or RNA must enter the cell; first it has to be absorbed, that the viral DNA or RNA penetrates the cell. For a short time were nothing appears to take place, then the replication of viral DNA or RNA and synthesis of other viral components takes place. During viral maturation the viral DNA and RNA and viral components are assembled. After maturation mature viruses are released from the host cell. Form of release varies depending on the virus type. In bacteria the cell is lysed and mature viruses are released. In higher organisms like man, the virus particles are extruded from the still living host cell. Most what we know about the interaction of viruses and bacteria are turning out to apply to higher organisms like man. The DNA in man is very complex and as such is providing other challenges in elucidating the interaction of viral DNA with human DNA. But, the results that will be described apply to humans. As we will see that bacterial DNA may also play a part in interaction with human DNA.

The process by which bacterial cells exchange genetic (DNA) material is called conjugation or recombination [5]. This was shown to take place in E. coli by Tatum and Lederberg long time ago. Two cultures of different mutants, differing in deficient genes was mixed together. The cells were isolated that were able to gain the needed genes from each other to eliminate the deficiency.

The process by which similar strains can gain genetic material that restores a specific capability is called transformation . The difference between conjugation and transformation is that in conjugation there is exchange of genetic information in living cells, while in transformation the living cell derives the genes from dead cells or free DNA.

The process by which a virus (bacteriophage) transfers genetic material to the bacterial cells called transduction. There are virulent phages and temperate phages and everything in between. Virulent phages as discussed before will cause death of the bacteria and release many phages. But, even in virulent phages, every millionth infection or so the virus does not produce many phages but becomes part of the bacterial cell. If this state the phage is called a prophage, and the cell with the prophage is in lysogenic conversion. The viral DNA or RNA can be integrated into the bacterial DNA (episome) or state as a separate unit of DNA in the cytoplasm (plasmid).

In addition there are temperate phages, phages that essentially can be used to transfer genetic material without lysing the infected cell. The bacteria can replicate with the phage DNA integrated or not. In that state, it is difficult to tell when a bacterium is lysogenized, without doing very sophisticated testing. But, occasionally the prophage leaves the host cell DNA and produces phages. So, the release of infectious phages in a culture is the best indicator that the cells are lysogenized.

Once the viral DNA is integrated, and gene of the integrated viral DNA codes for the synthesis of a protein repressor. This repressor protein is released in the bacterial cytoplasm and prevents synthesis of protein required for the lysis cycle.

As long as the repressor is synthesized, the phage is maintained as a prophage. If it stops due to "natural "or due to carcinogen induction takes place and complete lysis of the cell.. The repressor produced by a prophage prevents the infection of a lysogenized cell by the same phage that is carried by the lysogenic cell. The cell is "immune "to the infection by the same phage, but not against phages. There are also phages that are released in a lysogenic state that do not destroy the host cell.

Now let's review some of the significant consequences to bacteria being infected with bacteriophages that result in lysogenic conversion.

Streptococcus pyogenes causes infection of the throat. This bacterium is classified in-group A or Beta hemolytic Streptococcus. Bacteria are classified since there are many types. They are classified according to shape, size, producing spores or not, aerobic or anaerobic, fermentation patterns, and DNA analysis. Also on blood media this microbe will cause hydrolysis of the blood cells. This microbe in addition to causing impetigo or strep throat also can cause scarlet fever – red rashes on skin. This is due to the Streptococcus pyogenes being infected by a temperate bacteriophage that produces a toxin (erythrogenic toxin) that is absorbed into the bloodstream that carries a toxin to the skin resulting in a red rash.

Corynebacterium diphtheria causes diphtheria. These bacteria can synthesize the toxin that causes this disease only if it is lysogenized with a particular bacteriophage

Clostridium botulinum causes botulism, a killer toxin. Clostridium botulinum is an anaerobic, gram-positive, spore-forming rod. These bacteria produce A, B, C, D, E, and F toxins, each toxin is different. Here again, the toxin may be synthesized only by lysogenic strains of Clostridium botulinum. Each type of toxin requires different bacteriophage to establish lysogenic state.

Bacillus anthraces cause anthrax. The bacteria are an aerobic, spore forming, rod. The bacteria here also have to be infected by a bacteriophage to establish a lysogenic state to produce the toxin.

In all cases, when the lysogenic [prophage] is lost, the toxin production is also lost.

It is to be noted, viruses that cause cancer in animals may be defective viruses. Viruses that became lysogenized in animals first, then maybe become defective only in the sense that the virus has lost the ability to multiply and lyse the cell. In animal viral infections is more normal not to lyse the cell, but extrude the virus by enveloping the virus with part of the cell's outer membrane. It is suspected, that the cancer viruses have lost the ability to release viruses but are capable of expressing the viral genes in the cell. In the cell, due to repressor not active due to insults to the DNA portion of the virus that produces the repressor. It is also possible, as we will see later, that the virus reason unknown can be derepressed by insults to its DNA, and cause cancer as well as extrudes the virus. As stated before, it is possible, that in metastasis it is not the cells that break off from the cancer and establish a cancer colony at distal parts of the body, but the extruded viruses from the cancer cells that travel to distal parts and by infection of the distal cells cause the cells to become cancerous. The extruded virus most likely has all the inhibition sites destroyed as in the original cancer cell that produced the "defective" viruses. It follows that only cancers that can extrude viruses, can cause cancers at distal sites in the individual.

Interesting information concerning bacteriophage and bacteria is found in interaction off bacteriophage Mu and E. coli K 12 [2]. Bacteriophage Mu is a temperate phage. When E. coli K-12 are infected by phage Mu, about 2% of the lysogens are found to have acquired a new nutritional requirement. This unusual lysogeny caused the mutation and ergo the name Mu[mutator].

Most temperate phages integrate in one or a small number of specific sites in the host chromosome. Bu Mu can integrate into many sites. Mu DNA contains part or portion of host DNA. During lytic development, the phage DNA is associated with host DNA.

It also is interesting to note that those properties of phage Mu are similar to oncogenic animal viruses SV40 [Simeon virus 40] and polyoma as opposed to other Bacteriophages. Most lysogens contain only a single Mu prophage, but polylysogenic strains that contain two or more prophages, and at different sides of the host chromosome do exist. Mu is mutagenic in 1 to 3% of the lysogenic survivors. It appears that Mu induced mutations that are cause by linear insertion of the phage DNA directly into the gene and resulting in the gene being activated.

Mu can also cause deletion mutations. This phage can therefore integrate in many sites of the host DNA, in doing so it can disrupt gene functions. Also, multiple infections of Mu can occur, integrating at different sites on the host DNA, and not all of these sites are within genes, since many lysogenic states do not cause mutations.

From bacteriophage lambda we have learned that proteins produced by DNA of the prophage called repressor proteins turn off transcription [4]. In this way the repressor protein maintains the prophage integrated in the bacterial chromosome. If the repressor is inactivated the prophage becomes a phage and produces phages and lyses the bacterial cell. Various agents, including ultraviolet light causes the repressor protein to be inactivated. The mechanism of activation is not known, other than the agents change one or more of the DNA triplets which result in a protein that has one or more amino acids changed. The resulting protein does not bind to the receptor sites of DNA, by the very virus that the amino acid change prevents binding. But to be sure, other genes at the same time can be affected/changed and should cause problems for the prophage. Not being capable of mobilizing the production of necessary components to produce complete phages. That does not seem to take place, is still a mystery.

In all of the situations described, there are still many unknowns as well as known, and we are dealing with simple DNA of microbes not man. Man is many multiples more complex!

It is known that repressor controls the operator region and the promoter region on lambda prophage. The operator has three repressor binding sites. A promoter is a DNA segment necessary for binding off RNA polymerase and therefore for initiation of transcription.

There exists a bacteriophage in Streptococcus lactis bacteria that is used to produce cheese, buttermilk, and other fermented milk products [3]. When certain strains of Streptococcus lactis are treated with ethidium bromide the S. lactis becomes lactose and proteinase negative. When examined before and after ethidium bromide treatments, the S. lactis lost a 40 mega dalton plasmid. This inability to split lactose and protein hydrolysis, which occurs naturally at high frequency and is not reversible, suggests that these functions are borne by a plasmid.

Other plasmids were found also in some of the S lactis cells. But, the conclusion is that 40-mega Dalton plasmid was responsible for the loss of B-galactosidase[enzyme that hydrolyzes lactose] and protease activity

In this context, it is not so important whether this or that plasmid is responsible, it is important that a plasmid composed of DNA confers these properties, and in this case it is extra chromosomal. In the Streptococcus and Lactobacillus case the fermentation of lactose is important since the primary sugar in milk is lactose. Loss of this property prevents microbe from fermenting milk.

The genus Streptococcus also has some bad actors like S. Pneumoniae, S. pyogenes, and the flesh-eating Streptococcus. It is to date not determined if the streptococci have acquired DNA either by transformation, recombination, or transduction. But it is fair to say as these studies proceed that these dangerous properties are due to plasmids or episomes produced by transduction and lysogenic conversion. Note: the lactic streptococci [spherical] and lactobacilli [rods] effect the dairy industry and related industries. While the pathogens effect humans, dental caries, veterinary infections by_S. agalactis.

Further, in the area of toxin production by bacteria [1]. Many people have become deathly sick or die due to E.coli 0157: H7 toxin. It has been determined that these appears to be a similarity, if not identity between E.coli 0 157: H7 toxin and shiga toxin produced by Shigella dysenteriae type 1[a bacteria that is known to be pathogenic and toxin producing]. Therefore, there has to have been a genetic exchange between Shigella dysenteriae and E. coli to produce E. coli 0 157: H7 toxin strains. Was there a genetic exchange between two different genuses or is there a phage that infects both and becomes a prophage carrying the shiga toxin gene. There is also other good that comes from viruses infecting bacteria. Dr.A.M.chakrabarty with G. E. demonstrated that Pseudomonas [bacteria] that is capable of digesting octane and other octane like organic molecules from oil is capable due to plasmid that carries the genes for digestion. If the plasmid is lost, or it becomes lost due to the substrate depletion then the ability to digest hydrocarbons is also lost.

It takes some time for microbes to adopt [acquire capability to digest newly introduced substrates in their environment]. Take the oil spill in the golf, maybe, the loss of 75% or more oil unaccounted for is due to microbes adapting to the introduction of new substrates – oil into the environment, developing – acquiring the capabilities to utilize the new substrates – oil as food. Once the substrate – oil is utilize, the microbes are consumed by marine life as food, and there is nothing left of the oil.

Agrobacterium tumefaciens is a bacteria that causes crown gall [(a type of benign tumor in certain plants [7]. If the microbe is exposed to 37°C, the bacteria loses the ability to cause crown gall. This was shown to be due to the loss of a plasmid.

If the plasmid is reintroduced, the avirulent Agrobacterium tumefaciens becomes virulent. Crown gall is a malignancy affecting dicotyledonous plans. The plans can be infected by inoculating with virulent Agrobacterium tumefactions a wound site on the plan.

Note: DNA of several bacteria and animal viruses is circular. In other viruses as in all RNA viruses, nucleic acid is linear, but becomes circular immediately after it penetrates the host cell. How is this accomplished? Each single strand has a region at the end that is complementary to each other. They are joined by hydrogen bonds between complementary bases. The sugar – phosphate backbones are joined by enzyme called polynucleotide ligase, forming a fully covalent circle.

Note also: that circularity is also characteristic of bacterial chromosomes

The process of viral replication can be considered to take place in five steps

1. Entrance into the cell
2. Enzyme synthesis of viral nucleic acid.
3. Production of the viral components
4. Components brought together to form a complete virus.
5. Virus released from the cell, by the cell being dissolved.

If the viral nucleic acid is RNA, it serves directly as a messenger RNA. If the viral nucleic acid is DNA, it is first transcribed by a DNA dependent RNA polymerase to form viral messenger RNA. In both cases, the viral messenger is translated by host cell ribosomes to form enzymes necessary for viral replication as well as subunits of the viral capsids. The final stage in the reproductive process is the liberation of mature virions from the host cell. In animal cells this is often accomplished by extrusion through the cell membrane. In bacteria it is usually accomplished by lysis of the host cell through the action of viral enzymes

The host – range specificity of a virus is determined largely by the specificity of its binding to receptors sites on the host cell.

In every species of bacteria investigated for viruses, viruses have been found, also in blue-green algae and fungi.

Essentially a whole bacterial population may be destroyed in a few hours by phage infection by lysis. Chloroform kills bacteria but not viruses or phages. There is an interesting application of the knowledge of what causes bacterial destruction and knowledge of prophages. This is true in many industries, but specifically in the cheese processing industry from cow's milk. The microbe that is use to help cause the precipitation of milk proteins is Streptococcus lactis. S. lactis, like all microbes can be infected by variety of phages that cause lysis of Streptococcus lactis. This can be a total disaster to a cheese plant. In one day a plant can lose at least 100,000 pounds of milk to viral infection. And, the next day may be no different. To prevent this type of loss, the industry has produced many types of Streptococcus lactis that are infected by more than one bacteriophage and colonies selected that have become where the virus did not lyse the cell but becomes a prophase. This is done with as many as possible different viruses to cause the Streptococcus cells to become refractile to infection by viruses. Today, they can incorporate up to four different phages. This is not a permanent fix, since in time a phage appears that can infect the prophage containing culture of Streptococcus. Since there are now in stable state many streptococci cultures that have been caused to become refractile, these cultures are normally rotated weekly. Some cheese factories actually use more than one culture of refractile Streptococcus, but made refractile by different phages to give insurance.

Now, more about lysogeny. Following penetration of the bacterial outer membrane by the phage, the viral genome may be produced in synchrony with that of the host. The host survives and undergoes normal cell division to produce a clone of infected cells. In most of the progeny cells, no viral structural proteins are formed; most viral genes have been repressed. In an occasional cell however, derepression occurs spontaneously and the viral genome initiates cycle of development. In cells where this occurs, the cell lyses and liberates mature virionds.

Virus interacting with bacteria and not lysing the bacteria, the condition is called lysogeny [6]. The bacteriophage is called temperate phage in this situation. The genes in the bacterial cell of the virus are called prophage. Three processes are involved, 1. The viral genome is transcribed and translated to form the repressor molecules that inhibit viral replication. 2. Viral genomes is repressed. 3. The genomes enter the prophage state. Note: if viruses are produced before repressor action can interfere, the cell will be lysed. But, if the repressor molecules accumulate, viral replication is shut off and the virus becomes lysogenized.

Phage repressor molecules continued to be produced by the prophage and prevent viral production. Repressor molecules allow the replication of the prophage in the cell as the cell divides.

Note: my analysis

Once lysogeny takes place and the repressor molecules are produced and overtake the process, to prevent the virus going into the lytic state, the virus – host relationship is in steady equilibrium at perpetuity. But, if chemicals, environment, or whatever suppresses or destroys the process of repressor molecules being produced, cell goes into lysis. The cause of this is a change in the section of DNA [gene] of the virus DNA that produces the repressor molecules.

In cancer the repressed virus, repressed by repressor molecules that prevent cancer-causing virus from expressing, is stable and continues to either reproduce with the cell or is transferred to progeny. If the DNA of the virus that produces the repressor molecules is damaged, the virus starts to reproduce and destroys the cell and viruses are released into the bloodstream since by now the body recognizes the virus as non-self, if the original virus infection produced antibodies, the repressed viruses are eliminated from the blood stream, unless it is a progeny situation. In that case, there are no antibodies and can cause the disease. Now in cancer the repressed virus has to be damaged so that it cannot reproduce. But, if the repressor gene is also damaged, the virus then can cause cell to become cancerous, benign or invasive depending on the virus type. Cancer forms during our existence multiple times, but body's defense recognizes a non-self cell in most cases and destroys the cell – or cells and cancer potential is eliminated. It is in cases where the cancer cell somehow protects itself from being recognized that cancer starts, it eventually kills the individual. Unless during the Course of cancer treatment cells are "uncloaked" and recognized as non-self and destroyed.

Most of the original understanding we have of viral interaction is from bacterial cell [E. coli strain K 12] and from the action of bacteriophage lambda on that cell. The phage was discovered as a prophage presents in strain K 12 off E.coli. If a culture of strain K 12 is grown, few cells lyse and lamda viruses are released.

During cell division one of the daughter cells may not get lambda phage, and therefore that cell is cured of that phage. But, it can be infected by lambda phage, and the whole thing starts all over again – some daughter cells do not get the lambda phage. In both processes of conjugation and transduction, segments of the bacterial chromosome are transferred from one cell to another. The recipient has two sets of chromasomes,during the zygote growth into daughter cell; recombination takes place, which introduces new genetic material.

Note: when nonlysogenic donor cells were recombined with recipient cells harboring lambda prophage, the prophage was found to be inherited as though it occurred as a discrete site on the bacterial chromosome. Closely linked to the Gal. gene, which governs the production of the galactose utilization.

There is a gene in lambda that contains cohesive ends. There are single strands with complimentary base sequences, that allow the lambda DNA to close. Hydrogen bonding causes the lambda DNA to close. The circles are closed by enzyme called polynucleoside ligase. The integration of lambda into the bacterial chromosome is done by recombination enzymes, they cut the DNA molecules and rejoin the broken ends. This enzyme, on DNA structure, can cause the detachment of the prophage. The detachment of the prophage can cause the production of viruses from some cells.

So why not all of the prophages [lysogenic cells] go into production of viruses. Because, the integration of lambda with the bacterial chromosome requires the action of specific recombination enzymes, governed by lambda genes. The integration of lambda occurs before lambda repressor has had time to appear. Once it has appeared, however, it represses, all of lambda genes, including those for the specific recombination enzymes.

Therefore, the detachment is prevented, except in the rare cell in which the repressor is inactivated. What inactivates the production of repressor? Since the viral DNA segment produces the repressor protein, anything that changes that portion of DNA will cause the production of inactive repressor. Once the repressor is non-functional, sequence of events start to become lytic.

Another phage [P1] was also studied, and we have discovered more into the variety of functions of the P1 infection. It differs from lambda group of phages in two important respects. 1. The recombination experiments between lysogenic and non-lysogenic cells did not show chromosomal location for P1. 2. P1 and lambda are not the same in the incorporation of host DNA. Transducing particles of the P1 type may contain any host [bacterial] DNA . While lambda – only transduce those genes that are in the close proximity of its insertion. P1 type is a plasmid

In summary, a phage of the P1 type can replicates with the cell as a prophage, or go into the lytic cycle.

Lysogenized cells do not go into the lytic cycle due to phage repressor, not unlike in the lambda lysogeny.

In lambda virus, there is a gene [the Ci gene] that produces the repressor protein, therefore, there is a site on the lambda DNA that the repressor is bound to. If the site is not occupied by lambda DNA, the virus replicates. But, when repressor molecule binds to the DNA site, no gene expression.

Virulent mutants of temperate phage often occur due to the C-1 gene that was mutated so that the repressor is no longer produce, or the repressor does not bind to the receptor due to the change, or the receptor is altered and it does not attach. Some examples of conditions that can cause the virulent state are ultraviolet irradiation, temporary thymine starvation,

Mitomycin C treatment, or alkylating agents, just to mention a few

If a lysogenic cell allows other phages to be taken in – this is called super infection. If that takes place in the super infected state – there are three possibilities. 1. If this super infecting phage is resistant to the repressor produced by the lysogenic phage, the super infecting phage will multiply and lyse the cells. 2. If it is sensitive to the lysogenic phage repressor, the super infective phage will neither replicate nor express, and will be lost during multiplication of the bacterial cell. Virulent mutants [prophages that are resistant to its own repressor] will infect the bacterial cell and if also resistant to the lysogenic cell repressor will lyse the cell. Now, if the bacterial chromosome is mutated, so that no repressors are produced for phage infection/attachment, the bacterial cell is immune to the phage infection. Only phages that require that specific receptor sites on the bacterial cell surface infect. There are phages that have mutations in several genes, which prevent the phage from normal development. They can be detected by trying to infect with a co-immune phage, [phages that share sensitivity to the same repressor are co-immune] but, the co-immune phages do not infect, in most cases. But if they do infect and lyse the cell, some of the released phages are combinations of the two. Also, inducing agents can cause the prophage to reproduce.

In the super infected case, the defective phage can pick up the missing function[s] from the super infecting phage and become infective.

There are a number of bacteriophages that are strictly RNA based. When a RNA based virus infects a bacteria, the RNA is attached to the bacterial ribosomes. The combination somehow produced RNA which produce proteins. These are viral proteins that are used to produce new viruses. RNA viruses can also become lytic viruses by causing the cell to produce viral DNA by reverse transcription. The actual process by which this takes place is not known.

If the lytic virus in DNA form is caused to produce viruses, the viral DNA produces RNA, which is what the virus incorporates in the viruses. RNA directed the production of DNA, which directed the production of RNA. The RNA produced by DNA is the virus, or RNA virus.

Chapter 3, References.

1. Douglas L. Archer, E. coli o157:H7, Searching for Solutions, Food Technology, Oct. 2000, Vol. 54, No.10.

2. M.M. Howe and E.G. Bade, Molecular Biology of Bacteriophage Mue, Science, Vol. 190, Nov. 14, 1975

3. Steve A. Kuhl, L.D. Larsen, and L.L. McKay, Plasmid Profile of Lactose Negative and Proteinase Deficient Mutants of Streptococcus lactis C10,ML3, and M18, Applied and Environmental Microbiology, June, 1979, p. 1193.

4. M. Prashne, et al., Autoregulation and Function of a Repressor in Bacteriophage Lambda, Science, Vol. 196, Oct. 8, 1976.

5. Smith and Conant, Zinsser Microbiology, Twelfth Edition, 1960, published by Appleton Century Crofts.

6. Roger Y. Stanier, Michal Doudoroff and Edward A. Adelberg, The Microbial World, Prentice Hall, Inc., 1970

7. Bruce Watson, et al., Plasmid Required for Virulence of Agrobacterium tumefacience,J. of Bacteriology, June, p.255.

CHAPTER 4
VIRUSES TRANSFORMING
YEAST AND MOLDS.

SACCHAROMYCES CEREVISIEA A EUKARYOTIC microorganism, and its various subspecies and strains are used to make bread, beer, wine, whiskey, etc.[1]. The microbe uses the sugar in the various substrates to produce CO_2 and alcohol. The yeast uses sugar to produce ATP's – the energy source of life on this planet.

One of the strains of Saccharomyces cerevisiae is called a killer strain or strains. The killer strains contain two species of double stranded ribonucleic acid, one large and second small molecule.

Killer strains ability to kill sensitive strains and immunity against other killer strains has to contain the large and small molecule of extra chromosomal elements.

Not killer strains lack the small molecule of extra chromosomal elements, but some have the large molecule of extra chromosomal elements. These extra chromosomal elements are virus like particles.

Maintaining these two extra chromosomal elements that are RNA and are dependent on DNA for its maintenance. The killer strains produce a toxin that kills sensitive strains of all the yeast.

The reason that we are aware of this phenomenon is that in bread, wine [especially wine], etc. the final product did not result from the fermentation of the inoculated Saccharomyces cerevisiae. The reason after much research, it was determined that the yeast was destroyed by the killer yeast. Since this phenomenon was of interest to a large industry, research determined the cause.

It is very possible that like bacteria so yeast and higher organisms have various types of relationships with virus like or virus particles. Some of these relationships are good for survival like the killer yeast, other relationships are detrimental.

As we discussed in Chapter 3[in the cheese industry], the bacteria, if infected by viruses do not grow but are destroyed. That situation was of commercial interest, since if not solved, the whole industry goes out of business.

The bottom line, is that I am not aware of any situation be it bacterial or yeast that these type of perversions do not take place without viral interaction.

Chapter 4, References

1. Nieves Rodriquez – Cousino et al., A New Wine Saccharomyces cerevisiae Killer Toxin [klus], Encoded by a Double – Stranded Related to Related to a Chromosomal host Gene, Appl. Environ. Microbiol. March 77 [5], 2011, p.1822.

CHAPTER 5
HUMAN GENOME

AS STATED BEFORE, EVERYTHING we are is determined by DNA, but not the soul. The structure of DNA was derived by James Watson and Francis Crick in 1953 from data supplied by Rosalin Franklin. The molecule is a double helix and twisted ladder like. T is always linked with A, and G is always linked with C. The information DNA produces is produced by the atoms composing it, and the triple code for each amino acid was touched on in chapter 1.

For instance, in breast cancer a mutation in a gene on chromosome 17 [known as BRCA 1] causes cancer.

There has to be more to it than that. In light of the knowledge we have gained from viruses [bacteriophages] and bacteria, and to say that a single mutation or a change in one triplet is the cause of that cancer. That is hard to believe. It is more likely, that it is an indicator of something that takes place at the same time in the DNA, since not all mutations in a gene on chromosome 17 develop into cancer. It could be that a virus was absorbed during viral infection and integrated into one of the chromosomes, it becomes an episome, or the virus becomes part of the mitochondrial DNA. Note. The mitochondria have its own DNA and it is bacterial like double-stranded DNA.

Due to expanded developments in genetic engineering, it was decided to determine human genetic code completely [1]. Private funds were used at Celera headed by Greig Venter and public funds were used by the government to support the human genome project and headed by Francis Collins. Both organizations prepared drafts of their developments by 2,000. On the 50th anniversary of Watson and Crick's double helix publication, both organizations publically announced the results in 2003. They both together announced that the genetic code of humans was determined. Some of the interesting observations included, human genome DNA consists of 3.1 Billion single nucleotides on 24 chromosomes. They also determined that only 20,000 – 25, 000 proteins are coded by these genes. That accounts only for about 1.5 % of the DNA in humans. They also found that in insects, birds, simple plants and animals about the same amount of proteins are produced. So how do we humans are so much more complex. The simple answer is that we do not know. Since only 1.5% of human DNA accounts for the various proteins that we make and I presume need, what does the 98.5% of the DNA do? Is it accumulation of viruses and DNA that is shut off during differentiation?

In cystic fibrosis a deletion of just 3 nucleotides in the gene producing the necessary protein that becomes defective and does not function, causes the disease. This change is now referred to as DFTR. People that carry this defective gene can develop the disease. These changes can take place in X or Y chromosome. X is male and Y is female. If both X and Y is positive for this deletion, it will result in cystic fibrosis. But if only one is positive X or Y cystic fibrosis does not develop.

This is more believable, since in most likelihood it takes only a change in one protein to create the condition. It is not unlike what takes place in sickle cells anemia. A single mutation in the gene that produces the hemoglobin molecule that causes sickle cells anemia. To be more specific, the alpha chains are the same in normal and sickle cell anemia, but the beta chain in sickle cell has one amino acid that is different – instead of glutamic acid which has valine.

Note: for emphasis again, there are long stretches of DNA between genes that do not seem to be used for anything. Some researchers refer to these as "junk DNA". But based on our level of ignorance, that assumption is childish. These regions may be areas that the process of differentiation has shut off. Some of these areas may also harbor lysogenic viruses.

Assuming that the "junk DNA" harbors foreign DNA, it should be possible to determine in humans what foreign DNA is and where it came from. 1. By evaluating the genes by hydrolyzing the DNA into genes and then subjecting these genes to gel electrophoresis, and comparing numerous human DNAs, one should be able to determine DNA that is not common – ergo foreign DNA. 2. Comparing the foreign DNA [genes] with viral DNA [genes], bacterial DNA [genes] and yeast and mold, and maybe higher organisms, one should be able to determine were the foreign DNA came from – viral, bacterial, etc.

Through the ages, there must have been multiple viral infections like cold and flu, or H5N1 – avian flu, H1N1 – swine flu. As was indicated before, every one-millionth infection or so becomes part of the bacterial cell and most likely that also occurs in higher organisms, like man

The DNA operator – repressor system is probably operational in higher organisms like animals and man. Repressor molecule is produced by DNA directly and binds to DNA on specific sites of DNA called operators. This process of repressor protein when it binds to operator or operators prevents not only specific protein production, but also lysogenic viruses from expressing themselves.

A typical gene has about 1,000 nucleotides. The bacteriophage lambda contains about 50 genes, one of its genes is C 1 gene, and this gene produces the repressor molecules. It has been determined that that molecule is about 27,000 molecular weight.

Bacterial DNA consists of linear sequences, but DNA of eukaryotic cells contains many copies of the same DNA sequences and is circular. Note: one can isolate messenger RNA [m RNA] from the cytoplasm of cells and using the m RNA determine what portion of the DNA was transcribed when the mRNA was formed. The sequences in DNA that codes for say protein histone may be repeated 400 – 1200 times depending on the species. Some believe that this is how a lot or small amount are controlled for production. When you need more histone, you turn more histone coding signals on.

Plasmids transfer genes between species by picking up chromosomal genes from the host chromosome. This is not widely spread in nature. Plasmid engineering – uses plasmids to introduce foreign genes – called molecular cloning.

How is it done?

1. Break up the DNA into genes.
2. Separate the genes
3. Find a bacteria or virus that can be genetically manipulated
4. Introduce one or more genes in to this organism
5. Select the organism that has the inserted foreign genes.

As an example to further described the process of introducing foreign DNA into bacterial cells. A foreign DNA is spliced into a plasmid and introduced with the plasmid into a bacteria. First the plasmid is broken by the endonuclease Eco R1 and introduced into a single site that does not interfere with the plasmids genes for replication or resistance to say tetracycline. The tetracycline is a marker that will indicate that the bacteria have acquired the plasmid. The DNA sequence recognized by ECO R1 can be found in other DNA. ECO R1 one in every 400- to 16,000-nucleotide pairs and on a random basis cleaves the DNA. The fragments of choice are annealed to the plasmid DNA by hydrogen bonding and sealed by DNA ligase. The DNA that consists of the plasmid and foreign DNA are introduced into the bacteria by transformation. The foreign DNA is replicated with the plasmid. And you test to determine if the process was a success by subjecting the bacteria with the plasmid to tetracycline. If it survives the plasmid containing the foreign DNA is in the bacteria. Since one picks cells from colonies that started with a single cell, plasmid is duplicated during daughter cell formation.

By the way, to cause transformation to take place, the cells are subjected to calcium chloride treatment. The treatment makes the bacterial cell permeable to plasmids that can infect that particular bacterial cell.

In bacterial cells m RNA is made from DNA by transcription. Once the m RNA is made it goes to ribosomes to produce a specific protein. In mammalian cells during transcription, a RNA that is larger than m RNA is made and is called Hn RNA[heterogenous nuclear RNA]. Post transcription processes make m RNA from Hn RNA.

The protein specified by a gene itself i.e. its expression is regulated by the protein it produces. If there was no regulation, the various genes producing the various proteins would continue producing that particular protein – the consequence would be death. Therefore, it has been determined that the protein produced by a gene, itself is regulated. If the amount of the protein is approaching optimum, the protein throttles production of that specific protein.

Repeated segments of DNA in cells of higher organisms constitute a significant fraction of the genetic material. This can constitute one million identical or very similar copies. The origin and function of repetitive DNA still remains unknown. Other than another way of controlling overproduction of what that particular gene produces, and because that particular gene is important for survival, therefore there are more than one copy.

DNA was identified as genetic material in 1944. DNA structure was established in 1953. Replication, transcription, and translocation were established later. Repeating DNA sequences or multiple copies of the same or very similar base sequences was established much later. Repeating DNA copies have bin found in higher species that have been evaluated. In some as little as 20% and in others as much as 80% are repeating DNA sequences.

In cells of higher organisms, DNA reside in chromosomes. Chromosomes are nucleoprotein complexes composed of nucleic acid and proteins. Proteins function by maintaining the activity of the genes. Proteins control which genes are turned on and when. The control of genes is central of functions like differentiation and embryonic development.

Differentiation results ultimately in a cell types were only certain combinations of genes are transcribed or expressed in accordance with the cells specific functions. In bacteria binding and release of specific regulators at appropriate site on the DNA results in expression of a specific gene or not.

In cells of higher plants and animals the genetic material is more complex both structurally and functionally. The DNA is in a nucleus which is surrounded by a membrane. But, it still is the DNA that is the seat of inheritance.

In the nucleus, DNA is in contact with protein and some RNA to form chromatin and finally chromosomes. In higher organisms regulatory proteins have not been discovered. In bacteria regulatory protein have been demonstrated. The protein that DNA is associated with in the nucleus are histones and non – histones. The histones are positively charged, and contain basic amino acids. Histones are classified into 5 classes. They seem to be the regulatory protein. They are construction protein and by being construction protein, they prevent transcription into RNA. Therefore, they construct the chromatin and prevent RNA production.

The non – histone proteins are also involved with construction of chromatin. Both protein types are produced in the cytoplasm by mRNA attached to ribosomes. The non – histones are very heterogeneous or there are many of them. The non – histone proteins appear to be enzymes like polymerases – RNA and DNA synthesis and repair. Enzymes that work on other proteins, remove acetate, methyl, or phosphate groups.

If there are changes in non – histones, the consequence is changes in the cell, like the cell becomes cancerous. Actual results indicate that if a cell is infected with tumor viruses, there are changes in the histone proteins. These changes disappear if the virus becomes integrated into the DNA; otherwise, if the cell becomes cancerous, the changes in histones become permanent.

Chapter 5, References

1. Francis S. Collins, The language of God. Free press, 2006.

CHAPTER 6
INTRACELLULAR PARASITES.

IN THIS CHAPTER VARIOUS infections and not just viruses are explored, but viruses are also explored further. The indication is that not only viruses, but other DNA or RNA containing agents can transfer genes to the host.

First one is infections of cellular in nature, that is, infection inside the cell. We will look at examples of intracellular infections that change the cell.

One can look at intracellular parasites like Trichinella. It is a multicellular worm that invades the muscle cell. One can look at this infection like a virus that infects a bacterial cell.

Another example is a Protozoa like Leismania that a cell engulfs by a prokaryotic process. Heavily infected cells break down and liberate the Protozoa. Why the ingested parasites are not digested it is not known. It appears that the parasites are separated from the host cytoplasm by two membranes. When these parasites divide, its individual outer membrane surrounds each daughter cell. The membranes control the flow of material to the parasites. One form of Microsporidia a Protozoa causes encephalitis in mammals.

The H5N1 is an avian flu virus. NIH developed a DNA vaccine designed to prevent H5N1 avian influenza infection. This is based on modified version of the hemagglutinin[H] gene from that virus.

Pentagon implicated vaccine in death of an army SPC. The Army SPC received vaccinations for anthrax, smallpox, typhoid, hepatitis B and measles – mumps – rubella. The individual died a month after vaccination from symptoms that resembles Lupus, which is an autoimmune disease. It turned out that that individual had Lupus DNA markers. Some Lupus patients suffer side effects from vaccines made of live viruses such as smallpox.

How do viruses[RNA] produce their malignant effects [4]. Type C RNA tumor viruses produce several kinds of animal cancers. It appears they produce cancers by the process of transformation or a process by which normal cells become malignant – transformed cells. These cells multiply differently; they are locked in a more primitive state of development. How these transformations, come about is a mystery. Investigations have identified one and possibly more virus genes that is/are necessary for transformation. They also identified the proteins coded by gene[s].

Another striking aspect, several type C viruses increase their malignant potential by acquiring new genetic information from the cells they infect. Data from murine leukemia viruses shows that the genetic acquisition from host creates a slightly different virus, that is, each time the genetic transfer occurs. This led Richard Lerner of the Scripps Clinic and Research Foundation to conclude, that there must be a large number of viruses that cause leukemia.

It, for instance, has been shown that for avian sarcoma virus [ASV or Rous sarcoma virus] to cause cancer, the virus contains a gene [designated SRC for sarcoma] for a protein that has to be made, otherwise transformation will not take place. More important, investigators found that by examining fish to primates – they found that they all have one or at least very few DNA sequences related to the SRC gene. The gene has changed relatively little during evolution from fish to primates. Since this gene survived evolution, it probably has some function in normal cells.

Even in chemical induced tumors the gene produces the protein as in normal cells. Therefore, it may be that when the virus is a gene, the gene is change in some of the nucleotides and becomes transformed.

Researchers found that sarcoma virus originated from a virus that picked up SRC gene from the chicken cells and gained the ability to transform. Others have shown that murine leukemia virus do not themselves transform, but after serial infection of rats or mice with the leukemia virus and their reproduction in the animal – changed viruses are produced that can transform and cause sarcomas. Some researchers have found that only when leukemia virus exchanges one or more genes with another endogenous virus by recombination that the leukemia is produced in the mice. Some believe that even individual cases of mouse leukemia is caused by a slightly different virus.

There are many lymphoid cell lines from biopsies of Burkitt lymphoma patients [1]. These cell lines containing and maintain several copies of the Epstein – Barr virus [EBV] genome. There is a difference in the amount of EBV in the cells.

Some viruse's take cellular material from their host cell [5]. Most of the time the cellular material is glycoprotein or glycolipid. The purpose of the glycoprotein or glycolipid is to coat the virus and protect the virus from external factors.

Some RNA tumor viruses use glycolipids from host cell surface membrane to coat itself.

Rous Sarcoma virus causes sarcomas in chicken. The virus uses the transfer RNA of the infected cell as a primer for it's own RNA directed DNA polymerase [reverse transcriptase]. Without this enzyme the virus does not replicate nor can it cause cancer. The RNA of the virus is made into DNA by reverse transcriptase. RNA virus in DNA state is called a provirus. The provirus or in DNA form can produce RNA viruses. This RNA virus in DNA form can either exist as a separate entity or be inserted into the DNA of the host cell.

It is interesting to note, that so far studied RNA tumor viruses all have reverse transcriptase, but not all RNA viruses that contain reverse transcriptase are capable of causing cancer.

It has been stated that the genetic information for typeC tumor viruses resides in the DNA of the normal cells [9]. The virus can be activated by prolonged propagation in vitro exposure to x – irradiation on the halogenated pyrimidine derivatives, or inhibitors of protein synthesis. Once induced, one can see by electron microscope that the type C virions are present in extracellular space and budding from plasma membranes..

Another virus group includes small DNA containing viruses [8]. The following are typical Papova species: papiloma virus of man [common wart virus], papiloma virus of rabbits, Polyoma virus of mice, Vacuolating virus of monkeys [Simeon virus 40 or SV40, K virus of mice. Rabbit kidney vacuolating virus, and others.

The human wart virus is the first tumor-inducing virus that is active in cell – free preparations. That is, it can be isolated by filtering bacteria out of a solution containing the virus. The bacterial free solution will cause warts in humans by inoculation. The virus contains double stranded DNA. The virus, that causes warts, resides in the nucleus as inclusion bodies. The virus particles when they appear in the nucleus, they are associated with the nucleoli. If you look at cells in the wart, as you look from the skin to the top of the wart, you see the following. Cells first contain the inclusion bodies, then remnants of nucleoli and mature virus particles. Finally, the top cells contain only virus particles were the nucleus was.

It is oncogenic avian herpes virus that causes lymphoprolif-erative disease [6]. The vaccine that was developed is based on HVT [a new pathogenic herpes virus of turkeys]. This vaccine prevents cancer in chickens that become infected with Marek's disease virus [MDV]. This is the first vaccine that prevents cancer caused by MDV.

Today the MDV has become more virulent, and new vaccines are very helpful. Unfortunately, more strains are developing that are resistance even to the new vaccines. These new strains cause acute paralysis [the old strains cause transient paralysis], high mortality, with higher levels of lymph organ and skin pathology. To control the disease/cancer they are exploring DNA, that is, between birds with the disease and birds that are resistant, trying to determine which genes confers the trait of resistance. Also, at RNA level, they use DNA probes to identify genes that are different. To date, they found 3 genes that may be different. It seams that this virus can take on host genes or portion and become more resistant.

In bacteria the virus genes are integrated into the bacterial genes and reproduce along with the bacterial genes when cell division takes place. Each daughter cell receives at least one copy of the viral genes. How is that possible: 1. Viral DNA is inserted into the bacterial chromosome. 2. Viral DNA is separate from bacterial DNA, but replicates with the bacterial DNA. 3. Viral DNA replicates separately creating many copies.

We do not know if these same principles apply to higher organisms like man.

Example: As discussed before, K12 strain of E. coli has a provirus called bacteriophage lambda. Lambda inserts itself between galactose operon and the biotin operon.

FDA reported in 1973 that all the live virus vaccines are grossly contaminated with phages [2]. These bacteriophages are introduced into vaccines when viruses for the vaccine are grown in tissue culture. Bacteriophages are present in fetal bovine serum. The serum contains growth factors needed to grow cells in tissue culture. There are three possible effects: 1. We discussed the effects of various bacteriophages on bacteria. Some bacteria if infected by specific bacteriophage will either produce toxins or infect and cause disease. Examples are scarlet fever and diphtheria and there are others. There are many bacteriophages infecting bacteria that we are not aware of, since the combination does not produce any visible effects, again, as far as we know. 2. The second effect, it may be directed by the viruses interacting with the human cells directly by causing cancer or degenerative diseases. The interaction may be by these bacteriophages becoming plasmids or integrating into the human cell DNA. 3. It is known that some phages can reproduce in tissue culture. Can they replicate in cells in living organism like man. Millions of people have received live vaccines; there are no records as to increase in disease, or other melody that we know, and others that we do not know today.

Note: as smallpox virus genomes have been sequenced [3]. CDC and Russia has this information and possibly other countries. They have sequenced many types from many different countries. Cow Pox live virus has been used as vaccine. What effect or interaction does this virus have with the human cells besides preventing smallpox.

Microorganisms are ubiquitous, there is a book [7], Bergey's Manual of Determinative Bacteriology that just classifies bacteria, there are books classifying yeast and mold, and viruses. It is not surprising that microbes interact with humans or animals or other living systems. As stated before, even bacteria yeast and mold can be and are infected by viruses.

In man the various microbes live on the skin and in the intestinal tract. It is said, that there are more microbes in the intestinal tract then there are cells in the human body by a factor of about 1,000. The normal microbes inhabiting the surface of the skin and intestine are called normal flora. Others may be transient, and others may cause infections, disease and death. Many normal flora microbes may cause disease if given the opportunity – by acquiring genetic material that allows microbes to gain access or because the immune system is compromised. Even a microbe that inhabits the intestinal tract normally and represents up to 90% of the microbes in the intestine may become a pathogen if given an opportunity. Bacteroides, the microbes inhabiting the intestinal tract can cause septicemia or blood infection. If the infection is not treated the human may die. As in nature, competition is going on to become dominant on the human skin surface and in intestinal tract. If the wrong microbes gain dominance on parts or all of the skin – skin disease may develop from a rash to very serious. If the dominance is in the intestinal tract, you can have from loose bowels to bloody stool to death, if the dominant microbe invades the bloodstream and is not treated.

What is pathogenicity, or the ability by microbes to cause disease? It starts from their ability to change the structure and therefore function of the cells of the host or man. Therefore, there has to be interaction with DNA of the host. Here as with viruses, there may be residual affect on the host cell or cells that may manifest as aberrant growth of benign or cancerous tumor. This area of DNA interaction, change, and residual affect has not been studied.

Much what we know about human viruses has been deduced from viruses interacting with bacteria –bacteriophages. Note, Bacillecalmette –Guerin [BCG], it's an avirulent tubercle bacilli. Used as a live suspension to immunize against Mycobacterium tuberculosis [cause of tuberculosis]. This avirulent bacilli is very active in preventing tuberculosis by the individual being immunized against BCG.

In classification of viruses the following criteria are used: 1. DNA or RNA, single stranded or double stranded; 2. Viral structure helical, icosahedral, or complex; 3. Is the virus enveloped or naked; 4. Dimensions of the particle; 5. Immunology, cytopathology, or epidemiology. Classification allows everyone to speak and communicate about the same thing; unfortunately, classification does not cover the evolution of viruses, their process of infection, etc. Human beings love or hang on to classification as the end all. There are many things we should look at beyond classification. It is like when a disease is given a name, we know everything we need to know, but do we?

Besides the body defends against viruses by antibodies which act outside the cell to inactivate viruses, there is a intracellular agent or agents called interferon's. It is a protein induced by viral infections. It interferes with the replication of viruses within the cell. Once induced the interferon will act on other viral infections. There is a strong suspicion that double – stranded RNA initiates interferon production.

If a virus infects a cell and causes the cell to become cancerous, the process is called transformation. This is not to be confused with bacterial transformation. There are two types of tumors: 1. Benign – localize and not invasive into tissues or organs, and no secondary tumors produce. Benign tumors are completely removable by surgery. 2. Malignant tumors or cancers – invades normal tissue and organs and destroy them. Malignant tumor metastasis – cells or packaged viral particles separate from the main tumor, and travels to other parts of the body to form malignant tumors or cancers.

If cancer cells from one animal are transfers to another animal that is inbred, cancer may establish and grow. In not inbred animals, the cancer cells may be destroyed by immunity.

Early history of tumor virology.

Rous in 1911 found that sarcoma [cancer of the connective tissue] could be transplanted to other chicken. Shope in 1932 found that rabbit papilloma [wart like tumor of epidermal tissue] benign in wild cottontail rabbit, but causes carcinomas in domestic rabbits. Bittener a few years later found a specific virus in mice induces mammary gland carcinomas. The virus is transmitted from mother to progeny through the milk. Other viruses cause leukemia, solid tumors – lymphomas and sarcomas.

Virus – associated tumor induction [oncogenesis] facts.1. Long period between introduction of the virus and the appearance of tumors. 2. The disease [cancer] may be contagious – but the route of infection is not known. 3. Transformation efficiency is very low

Note: vast majority of viruses infected cells do not develop into cancer. Also, many animals infected with tumor viruses do not develop tumors. May be, in animals and not in tissue culture, many if not all do develop cancer, but the immune system recognizes the cancer cells and destroys the cells. The reason for resistance is not at all known, but most likely immunology plays a part. Only the cancer cells that can "Cloak" themselves from the immune response of the host develop into tumors – benign or malignant.

Note: Simian virus 40 [SV 40] discovered in cultures of Rhesus monkey kidney cells – used for growing large quantities of poliovirus.

Note: human adenoviruses [common in respiratory infections] could induce tumors in various rodents.

Rous sarcoma virus [RSV] in domestic fowl causes leukemia, and Rous virus produces sarcomas also. RSV is a part of a large group of viruses.

RSV is not a complete virus, and therefore, it needs a helper virus from the same group to be complete – therefore this is a two-virus infection. These viruses are all RNA viruses. Contact inhibition is a principal that involves all growing cells. When a cell contacts another cell, the cells stop growing or dividing to form two daughter cells. The normal cells grow in one layer – or monolayer. Transformed cells do not follow the monolayer principal or the contact inhibition principal. Cancer cells grow irregularly and form more than one layer.

The viral genome multiplies with the cell as the cell divides and the colony grows. In this case RNA is the viral genome and not DNA. Note: after the infection the RNA genomes are copied into DNA, and integrated with host DNA. This is accomplished via enzyme called RNA – dependent DNA polymerase. This enzyme does not exist in non-cancerous viruses. This enzyme is present in slow growing RNA viruses that may be involved in various nerve diseases. This enzyme is a useful tool to determine oncogenic virus infections.

Polyoma and SV 40 viruses. Both of these viruses are DNA tumor viruses. The DNA is circular and double stranded. If SV

40 is caused to infect green monkey kidney cells, these cells produce viruses. In human cells, the cells are transformed

Burkitt's lymphoma or mononucleosis in both, the most likely causative agent is Epstein –Barr [EB] virus that is also known as herpes virus.

Human breast cancer – is it of viral origin? Virus particles have been found in samples of human milk. These particles are virtually identical in structure to mouse mammalian tumor [Bittner] virus. Presence of these particles correlates with the incidence of breast cancer in families that have these virus particles. These particles contain RNA – dependent DNA polymerase. This is characteristic of animal tumor viruses

Approaches to determine that viruses cause human cancers. 1. Determine if viruses are in the tumor, and try to grow the virus in tissue culture to cause transformation. There may be drawbacks. Viruses are ubiquitous, and therefore may be only passengers. It could be that the whole virus cannot be found, but only some or all of viral genomes are present. 2. Test all known viruses for cancer by trying to transform human cells. Try to induce tumors in animals with the transforming viruses. FDA will not allow human testing. 3. Check for genes of known viruses in cancer cells. Use viral antigens or base sequence as genes for that virus. No human viruses that are suspected to cause cancer have been isolated. There are many isolations of genes from animals, and these genes are similar to genes isolated from humans. 4. Try to cause the virus to leave the cancer cell. Try the various methods that have been used to release viruses from animal cancer cells. Like U.V., drugs, and chemicals known to cause the release of viruses from animal cancer cells. But, mutations have caused the expression of the virus genomes as part of the DNA of the cell. The consequence of this is cancer. 5. Release of cryptic viruses from tumor cells by various means. This may be accomplished by irradiation, treatment with drugs, super infection with other viruses, or fusion of the tumor cells with another cell.

Chapter 6, References

1. Maria Andersson, Amount of Epstein – Barr Virus DNA in Somatic Cell hybrids Between Burkitt Lymphoma – Derived Cell Line, J. of Virology, Nov. 1975, p.1345
2. Gina Bari Colata, Phage in Live Virus Vaccines: Are They Harmful to People, Science, Vol. 187,Feb. 14, 1975, p. 522
3. Brian W. J. Mahy, at al., Sequencing the Small Poxvirus genome, ASM News, Vol. 57, No.11, 1991
4. Jean L. Marx, RNA Tumor Viruses: Getting a Handle on Transformation, Science, Vol. 199, Jan. 13, 1978.
5. Thomas H. Mauch II, Rous Srcoma Virus: A New Role for Transfer RNA, Science, Oct. 4, 1974.
6. Kyle S. MacLea and Hans H. Cheng, The Threat of Marek's Disease Virus is Expanding, Microbe, Vol.2, No.5, 2007.
7. E.W. Nester, C.E. Roberts, B. J. McCarthy and N.N. Pearsall, Microbiology, Molecules, Microbes, and Man, 1973, Published by Halt, Rinehart and Winston, Inc.
8. K.E.K. Rawson and B.W. J. Mahy, Human Papova [Wart] Virus, Bacteriological Reviews, June, 1967, p.110.
9. Sandra Panem, et al., Isolation of Type C Virions from a Normal Hunan Fibroblast Strain, Science, Vol. 189, June 25, 1975.

CHAPTER 7
HOW TO PREVENT CANCER

IN THIS CHAPTER THE various articles reviewed, should help further the understanding of viruses as the cause of cancer. It is also interesting to learn, that the mutations in DNA are caused by chemicals that are oxidizing agents. Throughout this chapter there are reviews how to negate the affects of oxidizing agents. The reviews to reduce the incidence of cancer are the reducing agents or antioxidants. Some vitamins act as antioxidants, some elements are also antioxidants, but the major antioxidants are found in plants. Plants use antioxidants to create no oxygen environment during photosynthesis. Photosynthesis does not work unless the environment is oxygen free. Some plant antioxidants are considered better antioxidants then others. The vegetable and animal fat industry uses synthetic antioxidants, which are touted as good for preventing cancer.

In final analysis, if the individual consumes variety of vegetables, antioxidant vitamins and antioxidant minerals, the chances of cancer are significantly reduced. That is the prevailing theory.

In this chapter as in the previous chapters, the articles selected are for illustration of the concepts of how to prevent cancer and not an exhaustive treatise of the subject.

There are two lines of cells in the lymph system [12]. There are initially no distinguishing characteristics in these cells. Hemopoietic stem cells are the precursors of the two cell types. The cell-derived immunity is responsible for initiating the immunity to cancer cells. With respect to the cells that produce antibodies, since there are many antigens in the environment, these cells respond to these antigens by producing antibodies. Antibodies are proteins and are found in the gamma – globulin portion of blood.

How was this information developed? It was done by examining people who lack one or the other or both cell types responsible for immunity. If the cells that provide immunity are missing, the person easily gets fungi or viral infections. In addition they have increase incidence of cancer. But, these people do not reject transplanted tissue or organs, if they live without getting fungal or viral infections. If the cells that produce antibodies are missing, these people get bacterial and also viral infections. If both cell type are missing, the person basically cannot resist any insults from the environment. If both are missing, it is found in children and the children die from essentially any environmental insult.

The antibody-mediated immunity is in animals associated with thymus gland. If the thymus gland is removed immunity is severally compromised. In chicken, production of antibodies is associated with lymph organ called Bursa of Fabricius.

Researchers found that in specific mice, if the thymus is removed, it somehow prevents lymphoma. This is the cancer of lymph tissue. Apparently, viruses can produce lymphomas only in lymph cells. Lymph cells source is the thymus.

Renato Dolbecco, Howard Martin Temin and David Baltimore were awarded the Nobel price in virology [39]. They discovered an enzyme they called RNA dependent RNA polymerase or transcriptase. Now it is known as RNA – dependent DNA polymerase also as RNA – directed DNA polymerase or RDDP.

The importance of this discovery is that RNA can be made into DNA. The theory was after the DNA discovery in cells and the alpha helix or DNA, that DNA makes RNA, and RNA makes proteins. The discovery of RNA viruses utilizing the RNA – dependent DNA polymerase the RNA viruses produce DNA. The DNA produced is a copy of the RNA in reverse. This is important to know since there are many RNA viruses that cause cancers in animals, and suspicion is that these viruses cause human cancers. At this time there is no conclusive proof. DNA and RNA cancer virus have been demonstrated in human cancers, but, since FDA does not permit infection by these viruses of humans, we therefore, have no direct proof.

In chickens if the bursa is removed, that also prevents lymphoma not unlike in specific mice. It is interesting to note, that the virus that causes lymphoma infects other cells in chicken. But, only if the bursa is present does lymphoma develop. These cells are continuously in a state of differentiation. Differentiation is the process by which germ cells like the immune system cells develop into cells that possess immune response. Therefore, it is the belief that cells have to be in the process of maturation – differentiation for the lymphoma virus to cause lymphoma.

It appears that antioxidants play a role in carcinogenesis. Vitamin C, Vitamin E and selenium were evaluated after treatment with carcinogens like dimethylbenz [a] anthracene [DMBA]. The reduction in cancers were between 15 – 50 % depending on antioxidant concentration. Butylated hydroxyanisole [BHT] and butilated hydroxytoluene [BHA] are used in preventing oxidation of polyunsaturated fatty acids in foods. Since these two antioxidants were introduced we have less stomach cancers. It also may be another reason. Heleco pulorii is a stomach inhabiting bacteria. It has been associated with ulcers, bleeding ulcers, and stomach cancers. Today, it is cured by derivative of penicillin. In the old days and still today use of drugs like tagamin still is used to control the growth of this microbe.

Critics of the carcinogen theory concluded that all compounds at some concentration and under certain conditions seem to cause cancer [30]. Therefore, the answer must lie elsewhere – with viruses.

Cancers or benign tumors were never found in long-lived animals on high antioxidant diets. The oncogenic [tumor causing gene] theory involves the activation of quiescent cancer genes by carcinogens, radiation or hormones to produce malignant cells.

It has been theorized, that cancer cells form throughout the life of an individual. The immune system recognizes that the cell has become a "non--self" cell and the immune system destroys it. Only if the immune system does not recognize the cancer cell as "non-self" that the benign or cancerous cell proliferates and establishes colonies at other sites [metastasis], and eventually the cancer destroys the individual. Or the benign tumor grows to appoint that it becomes necessary to excise the tumor. Since benign tumors are not cancerous – does not destroy adjacent tissue or metastasize – once excised, the individual survives unless the size of the tumor damages some vital system or organ beyond repair.

In the cancer case if intervention does not takes place, by radiation, and/or anti-cancer chemicals and/or surgery the individual succumbs to the cancer. In the situations where the individual recovers with the cancer even in five years not reoccurring, there are many reasons for the survival. The cancer was detected in the first stage – no metastasis and the cancer is completely removable by surgery without destroying a vital organ. In the situation where surgery does not remove completely the cancer or metastasis has taken place, the doctor is forced to revert to radiation and or anti-cancer drugs. In most cases that only extends the life span by couple of years. But in some cases the cancer disappears and the individual is cancer free for the rest of that individual's life, unless a different cancer develops and the whole process starts all over. How is the cancer disappearing possible, since it is not likely that radiation and/or anticancer drugs destroy every cancer cell. I believe, that in this case, the immune system recognizes the cancer cells – they had been "de-cloaked", and starts to destroy the cancer cells. In spite of the fact that radiation and anticancer drugs kill not only cancer cells, but also any dividing – growing cell, like immune cells, hair, and intestine columnar cells, etc.

There is a pill that cuts prostate cancer risk [33]. The drug is called Finasteride made by Merck and Company. Finasteride blocks the conversion of testosterone to hydrotestosterone. This is a hormone that all prostate cancers need to grow.

Of all the RNA viruses in nature, it was determined that retroviruses seem to be the only cancer inducing viruses[3]. From the RNA viruses it was determined that there are 2 polymerases, one is RNA polymerase the other is DNA polymerase.

Utilizing mengovirus, a picarnovirus and actinomycin D, There was no DNA activity, but production of RNA took place. It would appear that mangovirus has RNA – dependent RNA polymerase. That is O.K. for reproduction of the virus; it can produce the viral genome in RNA, and viral coat proteins.

But, for survival and longevity the RNA virus has to integrate into the DNA of the host. Utilizing the RNA dependent DNA polymerase, the virus RNA is made into DNA.

There seems to be integration of one or more types of retrovirus in most animal species. The fact that these retrovirus genes – virion, have not been lost, indicates that the virus genes are being used by the individual. Since through generations the virus was not lost.

The virus can be induced to leave the DNA and become a RNA virus, whether the viral DNA is lost or only used to make RNA virus that leave the cell by budding, it is not known.

Dulbecco and his colleges developed a test that allows them to test for viral DNA in a cancer cell [18]. The corollary must be also true – they can test non-cancer cell for absence of the viral DNA.

The possibility of getting cancer is inherited, except if it acquired during the lifetime of an individual [13].

Only one or few cells become cancerous, the others are not cancerous. If the cancer genes are inherited, they are in the other cells as well. If acquired during ones lifetime, the rest other than the cancerous cells most likely will not have the virus that causes the cancer, but they may have other cancer viruses not expressed. It is also possible, that the cancer virus, that is expressed, and acquired, is in other cells, but those cells just did not develop cancer.

Utilizing a new experimental approach, it was determined that SV40 genomes are found on chromosome No.17. It is possible that SV40 can be found on other chromosomes, but none were found.

Many other chromosomal changes have been found in cells that are cancerous. But, there are many cancers that do not have chromosomal changes. Therefore it is close to impossible to associate specific chromosomal changes with specific virus.

A tumor cell as it divides and the colony increases in size, it needs blood vessels to grow [19]. No blood vessels into the tumor no growth. To grow, the tumor releases a tumor angiogenesis factor [TAF] that vascularizes the tumor, and the tumor grows.

What is the chance that a cell will become cancerous? In a single adult, 4 million divide every second, 350 billion divide in a day, more than 10 to the 14 in a year. Also, there are about 600,000 new cancer cases in a year. This year, we have 215 million people; they produced about 10 to the 20th cells. Therefore, the possibility of a cell becoming cancerous is one in 10 to 17th. Cancer probably starts with a single cell; therefore, cancer is truly a rare event. Obviously, if one gets cancer the statistics are irrelevant.

Cartilage has no blood vessels. It was determined that cartilage produces a diffusible factor that prevents growth of blood vessels. Shark has no bones, just cartilage. Its cartilage was explored for control of blood vessel growth. The concept did not, in final analysis, prevent blood vessels growing into cancer colony.

To date, TAF has not been detected in normal tissue. No TAF has been isolated from regrowing tissue. If a tumor does not develop blood vessels, it does not grow. If the tumor develops blood vessels, it can send out cells to other parts of the body, to metastasize. The question still remains as to, be it the whole cells that are send out or only viruses, or virus like particles to establish cancer in other parts of the body.

Atherosclerosis is a disease of the blood vessels [4]. The disease narrows the vessel until it completely is closed. High levels of cholesterol are found in the plaque. This finding has caused the medical community to limit cholesterol in blood.

Some researchers believe the blood vessel disease is caused by a mutation in a smooth muscle cell, which grows into a benign tumor – the plaque.

There are 3 layers in the arterial wall – the intima, the media, and the adventitia. The inner surface is a layer of endothelial cells. Atherosclerosis takes place in the intima.

Before any carcinogen, virus, bacteria, etc. reaches the cells that the blood provides nutrition too, these carcinogens and invaders are in contact with the inner surface of the arteries. We know the effect on cells of carcinogens, and viruses. These carcinogens and viruses have the same effect on the cells lining the blood vessels.

During autopsy, the lesion consist of smooth muscle cells, macrophages, other white blood cells, connective tissue, blood protein, lipoproteins are found inside and outside of the cell, etc.

There are 3 theories of atherosclerosis.

1. Fatty substances get into the artery wall, as well as cholesterol that is an irritant.
2. Small clot is formed, that irritates the muscle cells. That irritation results in a plaque.
3. Single cell mutation takes place, it grows into a plaque. Stages in atherosclerosis. 1. Cell becomes cancerous. 2. Something promotes the cell growth. 3. Growth, dying, and breaking down.

Cigarette smoke is a good example of carcinogens, like benzopyrene and methylcholanthrene that are present in blood vessels in an individual that smokes.

Where did the virus come from? It is assumed that they developed from DNA of the bacteria into bacteriophages.it is considered also true for viruses that infect plants and animals [20]. It has been shown that bacteriophages interact with their bacterial host and can become lysogenized. At times one can find parts of the inserted viral DNA or RNA if it is an RNA virus, being released into the substrate.

Much of this information has been developed by hybridization of DNA in the cell or RNA in the cell with analog viruses.

It is also interesting to note, that RNA viruses come much later than DNA viruses in time.

It is also interesting to note, according to those authors, that they were able to cause 5 of the 6 RNA tumor viruses to be released from apparently normal cells. This would indicate that these viruses in DNA form are normally present in these apparently normal cells. Hybridization has been performed with RNA viruses, cancer viruses, and DNA viruses and found to hybridize. Therefore, these viruses are integrated into the DNA of the cell, and proven by hybridization experiments. Many of the animal viruses that cause cancer in animals have been found in humans by hybridization also. The simian RNA tumor virus has been detected in cells of human cancer patients. Under certain conditions these viruses are released from cells that are cancerous.

It would appear to me that what we are dealing with here is inherited viruses in lysogenic state. Under the right conditions, if the inhibitor protein is changed so that it does not react to prevent the virus from expressing itself. The normal form of expressing is the virus produces viruses. But, if some of the viral genes have been changed through the years, the virus is ineffective in producing viruses and takes over the cell, and the cell becomes cancerous.

This is the scenario with viruses that exist in a lysogenic state that is inherited.

Viruses that the individual acquires during ones existence and becomes integrated in some cells by lysogenic conversion can also either produce viruses or become cancer depending on how injured the viral genes are, and if the inhibitor is changed so it does not prevent the virus from expressing.

There are many natural compounds that can cause cancer [2], notably aflatoxin B produced by Aspergillus flavors. This is probably the most potent carcinogen known, Micrograms injected into a mouse can cause sarcomas. This compound is common in peanuts. Aflatoxin was a real problem for the Bontu tribe in Africa. The lowland tribe and the Highland tribe. both drank beer made at home, by molding grain first then followed by yeast fermentation. The molding or growing mold on the grain produce aflatoxin B. Both the low land and the high land drank that beer contaminated with aflatoxin B. In addition the low land beer drinkers were infected with the virus that causes hepatitis. That combination in the low land men produced liver cancers. In US people who had hepatitis are warned not to drink alcohol, since that combination also can produce liver cancers.

People in Japan, in the past made their own soy sauce at home. Japanese were known to have high incidence of stomach cancer. Since today most soy sauce is made in plants like Kikoman, the incidence of stomach cancers are significantly lower. Soy sauce production also first includes molding the grain and then fermenting the molded grain in 18% salt solution. The molding step if not controlled can be contaminated with Aspergillus flavors and produce aflatoxin B. It is impossible to determine with the naked eye if the molding grain contains the aflatoxin producing strain of Aspergillus, since the normal Aspergillus used to mold the grain is identical to the toxin producer by the naked eye.

As stated before it may take 10 to 20 years for cancer to develop.

The carcinogens are detoxified by mixed function oxidases. These are enzymes that metabolize various exogenous chemicals and drugs and make them harmless to the animal or human, but not all. Example of a carcinogen that becomes more carcinogenic is aflatoxins, and there are others that we know and others that we do not know at this time. These enzymes are in the liver.

Also, besides asbestos and arsenic many metals or their salts cause cancer like beryllium salts, cadmium, or cadmium sulfate, Nickel, cobalt, chromium, lead as pure metal, it salts, or the ore. Asbestos causes mesotheliomas [originating from cells of epithelium lining internal body cavities]. Combination of two or more carcinogens can cause cancer, even though each individually has no affect due to low dose. Non-carcinogens can increase the carcinogen toxicity in its actions.

Note: certain chemicals can act as promoters that are themselves not carcinogenic, can increase the activity of weak carcinogens or of minute doses of strong carcinogens. All carcinogens are known as initiators of cancer. Initiated cancer may stay in that state for years, and if a promoter promotes or some other not known event takes place, this can result in cancer.

In healthy individuals the immune system keeps the emergence of tumor cells in check. Interferons are specific proteins synthesized in certain cells that inactivates viruses and are implicated in preventing tumor cells from developing or destroying developed tumor cells.

Nobel laureate Has Gobind Kharana from MIT synthesized a gene that correct a mutation defect in bacteriophage lambda [29]. The synthetic gene is 207 nucleotides long. This gene codes for tyrosine transfer RNA.

It is a known fact, that majority of all cancers are caused by the environment and therefore preventable [34]. Reduction of cancer should be as simple as getting rid of carcinogens from the environment. But there are problems, 1. Cause and effect has not been conclusively established. Nitrates lead to nitrosamines that cause cancer, estrogens, saccharine, and promiscuous sexual intercourse can cause cervical cancer, most likely due to herpes virus infections, 2. We cannot exist without some carcinogens. 3. Public resistance. DeLaney amendment – no food or food additive that was shown by DeLaney to be mutagenic and therefore, assumed to be carcinogenic at any level, cannot be sold in California. Thank God, it was not implemented nationally, since an amino acid critical to human existence at certain concentration causes mutation of the Salmonella that is used for these tests.

Epidemiologists have determined that a large proportion of cancers are caused by the environment [24]. So, Bruce Ames of University of California, Berkeley has developed a simple system for taking a quick look at the mutagens, and by inference carcinogens. To test a chemical for carcinogenesis by the official method in lab animals takes 2 to 3 years and costs at least $250,000 per chemical. Ames test uses Salmonella typhimurium histidine negative which is a bacteria. The test includes growing bacteria in the presence of a particular chemical at various concentrations. After the chemical exposure, the bacteria are tested for histidine. If the bacteria gained the ability to make histidine, it is considered a carcinogen. Growing on histidine free media indicates that the microbe now can make histidine. By this method it was determined that 156 out of 174 or 90% known carcinogens cause mutations in Ames bacterial strains. Very few of the 109 "none carcinogens "tested cause mutagenesis.

In prostate tumors there are biochemical markers in blood [5]. In other cancers there are other biochemical markers. If these biochemical markers are released into the blood by that cancer cells they can be tested for, if they are unique to the cancer cells. We will discuss in the next chapter the significance and how to take advantage of this knowledge in curing cancer

During World War II – they used chicken embryos to produce yellow fever vaccine [40]. In the vaccine most likely was a virus that causes neoplasia in avian species. The question was, can this virus cause leucosis or sarcoma in humans. They studied World War II veterans. Avian viruses have seldom induced neoplasia in mammals, except for Raus sarcoma virus, which can induce sarcomas in mammals.

More than a third of World War II veterans receive yellow fever vaccine but only small percentage died of cancers after 20 years. They looked in 1952 – 1954 and 1959 – 1963 death certificates off World War II vets. This is a very small number of humans dying from cancer. This may have been due to the neoplasia virus providing immunity from cancer and not causing cancer in humans.

Murine sarcoma virus hybridization test show large amounts of virus – specific RNA in the nucleus and cytoplasm of virus producing rat and mouse cells transformed by murine sarcoma virus [MSV] [38].

It was not a fact in 1972 that viruses cause human cancer [15]. Reverse transcriptase or RNA – directed DNA polymerase was discovered. And, it became known that most viruses known to cause cancer in animals are RNA viruses. In 1972 there were two RNA cancer virus theories. 1. Provirus or RNA tumor viruses infect a cell. The RNA is via RNA directed DNA polymerase copies itself into the DNA, and it comes an oncogenic virus. This causes normal cells to become cancerous. 2. This hypothesis states that the genetic information for cancer already exists in every cell. It is transferred genetically from parents to offsprings. The RNA viruses infected years ago. The virus is prevented from expressing. When it starts to express due to environment, it can cause cancer. If a cell becomes cancerous, cancer virus may not be found. If no viruses are produced after cancer develops, it may be that the virus has been activated but it has lost the ability to reproduce. So, it uses the cell to do its dirty work.

Raus sarcoma virus induces tumors in chickens, which put forth the hypothesis that viruses cause cancers. Breast cancer, leukemias, lymphomas, sarcomas hybridization experiments have shown hybridization to Raus sarcoma virus. Therefore, there is a relationship between the cancer mouse virus and the genes in human cancer cells.

Note: in many leukemia patients, reverse transcriptase is present in association with a high molecular weight RNA. The RNA is the RNA of Raucher leukemia virus.

There are three requirements to link RNA tumor viruses to cancer. 1. High molecular weight RNA in cytoplasm. 2. Reverse transcriptase is present. 3. The genes in the cancer cell are found in cancer virus.

Many investigators caused normal healthy cells to release viruses by chemical agents that cause mutations. To date, reinfection and producing cancer has not been done.

Note: Infection of susceptible cells by the cancer virus can take place if no repressors are present. This may happen in inbred animals. You do not see this in nature, if you did, cancer would be an epidemic disease.

Injection of inactivated type C RNA viral vaccine reduces the incidence of sarcomas [41]. The chemical use was 3 –methylcholanthrene. Type C RNA virus reduced but not completely prevented sarcomas.

It is assumed, that when cancer genes are turned on by outside agents, the cell becomes malignant and grows into a tumor [32]. It is also probably true, that benign tumors follow the same process. Therefore, one can assume that benign or malignant cancers are inherited. Chemicals, radiation and hormones bring out the cancers. In many cases no viruses are detected when the cell become cancerous, only markers of these viruses, such as antigens or reverse transcriptase appears. Therefore, there is only partial expression of a virus, and the complete virus does not have all the components to become a virus. But, the components of the viral DNA that are expressed cause the cell to become cancerous.

Note: This article addresses cancer viruses that is received from parents, but not acquired during life of the animal.

Retroviruses are RNA viruses that have the ability to become provirus [11]. These viruses are very carcinogenic. These viruses can cause cancer in relatively short time in animals like chicken, turkeys, mice, rats, cats and monkeys. These viruses have genes for cancer and genes for producing new viruses.

It is possible to incorporate eukaryotic DNA genes into other eukaryotic cells; this usually is accomplished by calcium phosphate precipitate.

It is also possible to enzymatically chop up the DNA of viruses or cell DNA and cause transformation of cells.

It is assumed that since so called normal cells contain genes that can transform regular cells. The activity of these genes introduced into normal cells can be detected.

Here again there is a strong indication that these transforming genes are inherited, maybe generations ago. By fragmenting the DNA into genes, the inhibitor for viral expression may be lost and also the genes for producing new viruses. As a consequence, the virus genes that transform produces cancer. Since, the virus has no capability of being integrated into the DNA of the cell due to loss of inhibitor and also, the loss of the ability to reproduce.

So-called normal cellular genes have been looked at that may have cancerous activity. And, at least in some cases, the expression of these genes can cause cancer. There seems to be dominance by the transforming genes that cause cancer. It would appear that there are specific pathways of oncogenesis. It would appear that the pathways are like the discrete stages of lymphocyte differentiation

The transforming genes of human bladder and lung cancers have been identified by homology to the rat genes of Harvey and Kirsten sarcoma viruses. Molecular cloning of these genes has been accomplished in some cases.

In this article, I did not see any comparison of normal cell DNA with cancer cell DNA. It would appear to me, that if the comparison were made, the genes in question would be found only in the process of being transformed to a state of transformation.

It is also interesting to note, that in this article they used a process of identifying active from inactive genes. This is very important for the proposed process later in this book . This will be needed to identify the specific genes of cancer cell and compare it to normal cell genes that are expressed.

Note, as stated before, the normal cell may harbor the transforming viral genes received from parents or the virus is acquired during infection of the individual during a lifetime.

If the cancer virus was received from parents, analysis of the total gene pool of normal cell versus cancer cell will show no difference in the genes. The only way to determine the different genes used by normal cell and cancer cell is to examine the active genes only. In which case there should be a difference. The different genes in cancer cell as compared to normal cell will be the cancer genes.

In the case of virus that cause cancer acquired during the individuals lifetime, one can compare either the expressed genes or total genes to find difference in the type of genes. If you find no difference in the total genes analyzed, then one is dealing with viruses acquired from parents, or the normal cell chosen is a cell that contains the virus in a steady acquired state. One should evaluate other cells from the same organ for the identification of cancer specific genes.

Rous sarcoma virus transforms chicken fibroblasts. This RNA virus has a gene, a single gene that transforms. This gene is not needed for viral replication. This RNA virus when integrated into DNA, it does so at a unique site on the DNA. This can be prevented from producing the end product that transforms the cell by an inhibitor. But, if the repressor, which is produced by DNA, is missing or the DNA that produces the repressor is damaged and produces inactive repressor. If the gene is then transcribed, it produces its end product that transforms the cell. This virus can produce viruses while transforming the cell.

The transforming RNA viruses run the gamut of affects. Some, like Rous sarcoma virus transforms quickly infected cells, it also transforms cell lines. Others transform the susceptible cells in living being, but not that same cell line outside the lining body.

Other take a long time to transform, some not in the study period.

DNA viruses transform small percentage of cells. The estimate is one in a 100,00. But; the results of the transformed cell are highly transformed to barely transformed. Also, the viral DNA when integrated into the cell DNA is highly controlled. The cell DNA does not permit the viral complete expression that would result in cell death. Also it appears that transformation is not independent action of DNA viruses like RNA viruses. Transformation is linked to viral production.

Families of viruses that infect vertebrate [35].

RNA DNA
Arenaviridae Adenviridae
Bunyviridae Herpetoviridae
Coronaviridae Iridoviridae
Orthomyxoviridae Papovaviridae
Paramuxoviridae Parvoviridae
Picarnaviridae Poxviridae
Reoviridae
Retroviridae
Rhabdoviridae
Togaviridae

Members of the following families can cause cancer: Retroviridae, Herpetoviridae, Adenoviridae, and Papovaviridae. Poxviridae viruses, some members may cause benign tumors.

Chemicals that react with nucleic acid initiate tumors. Initiation, it would appear not to be reversible, but, by itself does not produce cancer.

You need chemicals that promote the initiated cells to form cancer cells. Transformation is very low in chemically induced cancers, unlike viral cancers. Even, less than DNA viruses in living systems.

Every tumor produced by chemicals produces different antigens, which do not cross react. Virally induced cancers produce antigens that correlate with specific virus.

Chemicals that cause cancer in animals, these same chemicals cause cancer in man. This is in man by inference, since no experiment has been allowed to try to produce cancer in man by cancer inducing chemicals.

Same applies with viruses. Viruses are well established as agents of cancer in animals. There is to date no proof that cancers are caused by viruses in man. Hybridization experiments have proven conclusively that viruses are present in the DNA of animals. But, no such information is available in man. The government via FDA would not allow doing experiments with viruses in man.

Cancer is mostly an old age disease [8]. One can classify cancers by type and organ affected. By type, we are dealing with epithelial cells that include the skin and glands and are called carcinomas. If cancer develops in fibrous tissue or blood vessels, these are known as sarcomas. The third group includes blood and lymph system and are known as leukemias or lymphomas respectively.

If one classifies cancers by the organ they are found in, which includes many dissimilar cancers. Since there are many types of cancers classified by type of organ, it has to be assumed that there are many causes. But, no matter how many causes, they all start and continue via DNA.

It would appear that as previously stated, cancer is unavoidable. Cancer can be looked at as some cells become cancerous, these may survive for some time, but the immune system recognizes them as non-self and destroys them. Others may grow into small colonies, and be also destroyed by immune system, or may exist for some time or until the death of the being from other causes. The cancers that do survive and grow, that become a problem and need treatment, as we stated before, these need to be induced and then promoted to cause cancer. Inducers and promoters, some are known others are not. And, we may be introducing inducers or promoters through chemistry continuously. All of our carcinogens are tested with animals. Animals have short lives, and we make the assumption that we can correlate their time of cancer appearance that in man can be 90+ years. But, can we make that assumption; of course that has been the premise.

We do not know with certainty when the induction and promotion takes place. From animal experiments we calculate it to be 10 – 30 years. Some indication from cigarette smoke and cancer. Some have smoked until about 10 – 15 years ago and stopped. Some develop cancer, but not all.

Is environment involved in causing cancer? There are many groups of people studied, as well as migration of people. For Example, in Japan stomach cancers are much more prevalent then say in U.S. But, if Japanese migrate to U.S., this cancer decreases in a generation. Today. We think we know what caused it. We discussed this before. It was to do with soy sauce manufacture. Japanese use a lot of soy sauce. Then it was made at home, and today it is made in plants that control the process. The home brewed sauce in many cases contained Aflatoxins, a powerful carcinogen. This carcinogen is suspected as the cause of stomach cancer.

In U.S. the soy sauce is made in plants not at home. Stomach cancers are lower. But, if Aflatoxins were the cause of stomach cancers in Japan, then, why do they have a lower incidence of cancer of the large intestine. Aflatoxins are one of the most carcinogenic substances in the world, and some of them must have ended up in the small and large intestine. Why lower incidence of large intestine cancers in Japan? Later it was proposed that in Japan the intestinal throuput is faster due to consumption of vegetables they consume. The throuput in U.S. is much lower. Later it was discovered that microbes in the intestinal track can convert cholesterol into cancer inducing chemicals, if given the time to do so.

By the way, any animal of any age will produce a cancer if given the right chemical carcinogen by almost any route.

Metastasis – the spreading of the cancer to other parts of the body.

Inherited DNA defects can also cause cancer. If one has poor DNA repair enzyme, skin cancer can develop, Skin cancer is more relevant in those people, but not all. Many other genetic situations are known that should result in cancer, but they do not.

We know today that lung cancer is caused mostly by cigarette smoke. Not all that smoke get cancers, even though lung cancer is on decrease in men – in women it is on the increase, and it is assumed that that is due to the fact that women took up smoking while men decreased.

Cancer of the stomach has decreased dramatically in U.S. Factors that have caused the decrease are unknown completely. There are two factors that are known. One, aflatoxin production in peanuts. Since this was discovered, the aflatoxin in peanuts is being controlled. The other, the microbe that inhabits some stomachs is H. pulori. This microbe produces ulcers; there are indications that this microbe also can cause cancer of the stomach.

Cancer of the large intestine is associated more with rich countries than poor countries, as stated before, this can be due to food consumed and the effect of the bacteria in the large intestine that can produce carcinogens from certain ingredients in food. High Cholesterol diet in rich counties may be the culprit.

Virus causing animal and human cancers have been investigated. In animals, the cancers have been investigated, and viruses were found. The animals can be infected and the virus produces cancer. It is not so clean in humans. Animal viruses that cause cancer have been isolated from cancer cells. Cell lines can be infected by the isolated virus, and the cells become cancerous. No human has so far been injected with cancer virus to determine cause and affect.

Is the human cancer virus real? Since, to induce cancer by any means including viruses is prohibited by law, it is impossible to answer that question [9]. But, viruses as causing agents have been implied. For example, Epstein Barr virus has been isolated from infectious mononucleosis and Burkitt's lymphoma. Also, Burkitt's lymphoma appears, not always, in individuals that had infectious mononucleosis. Individuals that do not take care of themselves after infectious mononucleosis, but not always. Not taking care of yourself after infectious mononucleosis is not a predictor of Burkitt's lymphoma. As stated before, no studies in individuals with these viruses has been done. Viruses have been isolated often from infections. Therefore, no cause-and-effect has been demonstrated.

Systemic lupus erythematosus [SLE or lupus] and related conditions [affecting about 500,000 people yearly] and rheumatoid arthritis [affecting about 5 million persons] are autoimmune diseases [28]. Immune system protects against bacterial infections, viral infections and possibly tumor cells. In the autoimmune disease state the immune system attacks the body's own tissue. In rheumatoid arthritis the joints are attacked. In SLE, immune system may attack any organ or systems,

Immune system is responsible to detect and destroy damaged cells, viruses, bacteria, and cancer cells. The detection information is on the surface of the cell that is to be destroyed. It is assumed, that the surface of cancer cell should be different than normal cell; but, maybe not so different as to come to the attention of the immune system. If nothing else than the contact inhibition system should be detected, but obviously it is not. Even though, the cancer cells are not subjected to contact inhibition. And that also is not detected by the immune system.

As previously discussed, it is possible that since viruses are released by cancer cells, and therefore, not cancer cells but viruses or viral particles are the cause of metastasis. Cancer metastasis is not random; the metastasis takes place from specific organ to specific organs. This indicates viral and not cell metastasis. Therefore, this ability to grow in foreign sites is not a universal property of cancer. Basal cell carcinoma and brain cancers do not metastasize as a rule. Some can produce metastasis before the original cancer is detected. This strongly indicates viral not cell metastasis.

In SLE disease anti DNA antibodies were found in blood. Investigator found SLE associated with C type virus, which is a RNA virus. This virus produces cancers in mammals and chicken. The autoimmunity may be due to the fact that the virus altars one or more surface proteins [antigens] enough to cause the cell to be non self. This immune system recognizes this cell[s] as non-self and starts to destroy them. This condition or these cells are a form of cancer. The cells that are being destroyed may be cancerous. These cells are on the way of becoming cancerous, but first these cells change the surface antigens. Like the contact inhibition proteins.

There is numerous evidence that RNA viruses are associated with SLE

These diseases effect more females than males, and these diseases are more serious in females as a generality. SLE can also be devastating in males. They suspect that female sex hormones have an affect on regulating T – cell antibody response to RNA and DNA viruses. Male sex hormones seem to somehow have the reverse affect. In addition, in SLE, susceptibility to viruses, and defect in immunity may also be involved.

Sunlight causes 25% of all malignant lesions [22]. Squamous cell carcinomas are directly caused by chronic sunlight exposure.

RNA retroviruses move in and out of chromosomes with considerable ease, they tend to select genes for proteins that "have key roles in cell growth and control" [16]. They may sometimes cause recognizable disruptions leading to malignancies. It is strongly suspected that RNA retroviruses cause cancer in humans. Papillomavirus and hepatitis B virus [H BV] also is suspect in human cancers.

Primary bone sarcomas of the dog and cat the majority are osteosarcoma [1]. The other sarcomas include: chondrosarcoma, fibrosarcoma, hemongiosarcoma, liposarcoma, undifferentiated sarcoma, it's DNA or resulting product of the bacterial DNA causes a "virus" to become active.

National Cancer Institute is developing vaccines that should prevent cancer in man [25]. Vaccine is being developed against herpes 2 virus, that causes cervical cancer. This is prevention and not a cure. They are also working on a vaccine that will prevent lung cancer. Again, this is also prevention and not a cure. It does indicate, that specific viruses cause these cancers. It also indicates, that by producing antibodies against these specific viruses, the virus is prevented from infecting the cells to cause cancer.

Vaccine against hepatitis B and liver cancer is also being developed. This again is preventive against viral infection and not a cure if the cancer is there already.

Antituberculosis vaccine is being developed or BCG. This vaccine appears to work against leukemia, the leukemia that is common in children. This vaccine is preventive and nor a cure.

They found that if mice or rats are heavily injected with cancer cells from cancer animals or cancer viruses, they produced immunity in those mice and rats.

Next, they decided to infect other animals with cancer cells from cancer animals. They have seen remarkable results with these animals. FDA has prevented this type or research with humans.

This process works on induced as well as spontaneous tumors. Once immunity is established in the susceptible animal, that immunity prevents other types of cancers. Therefore, there exist commonality in cancers.

Studies in rats showed that immunized mothers transmit protection through breast milk and across the placental barrier [23]. 100% of offspring survive lethal doses of Gross leukemia virus. Cancer was eliminated in infants by immunizing their mothers with injections of Gross leukemia virus. A single injection of 0.01% of Gross virus was found to yield lethal leukemia in all rats younger than two weeks of age. You cannot Immunize the young rats since they do not have a developed immune system. The hope was that the mother will passively transmit the immunity to their offspring after the mothers are immunized

In 1971 Arthor S. Fleming award was presented to Harvey Graham Purchase for the study of leukemia known as Marek's disease, a cancer of chickens [31]. His studies resulted in a safe and effective vaccine. First vaccine against cancer. Now, how does this apply to human cancers. Burkitt's lymphoma is similar type of cancer in man . We do not know at this time the potential outcome, since studies of this nature are not permitted by the governments of the world.

Today cancer treatments include drugs, x-ray, and surgery [17]. These treatments can at times induce antibodies with corresponding total regression due to immunity. In most cases these treatments only prolong life, and finally the patient succumbs to the cancer.

They found that RNA from lymphocytes from animals that had cancer of polyoma virus, had RNA that prevented cancer. Taken these lymphocytes and mixing them with the cancer cells destroyed the cancer cells.

They fractionated the active RNA, which represented about 5% of the total RNA. They tested all fractions of RNA. Mixing this active RNA with human white blood cells, caused the human white blood cells to attack the animal tumor cells, in the test tube.

Therefore, animal RNA from a cancer animal can confer immunity to human cells.

Grape seed extract is a powerful antioxidant [26]. It is better than ascorbic acid or tocopherol .

Coenzyme Q 10 key role is in producing ATPs [10]. ATP is the energy of life. Coenzyme Q 10 also functions as a powerful antioxidant. It occurs widely in food supply, cells do manufacture coenzyme Q 10. This enzyme was discovered in 1957. This enzyme is helpful in cancer prevention, probably as an antioxidant.

Research indicates that conjugated linoleic acid [CLA] helps fight cancer [37]. In 1978 Michael Pariza Ph.D. took nine years to isolate the CLA. He published his results in 1987. CLA is found in fried foods, milk products, oil of safflower, and other foods. The c9t11 isomer seems to be involved in preventing cancer. Possibly benefiting in all three stages of cancer – initiation, promotion, and metastasis. The typical commercial isomer mixture appears to be the best isomer ratio for cancer prevention.

Dr. Pariza started with the Food research institute after receiving his Ph.D. from MIT. Right around the time he started, it was discovered that fried food, like hamburgers, during frying produces benzo-A-pyrene, not unlike cigarette smoke. Benzo-A-pyrene is one of the most carcinogenic compounds found. He studied the problem extensively. Initially he found that extract of cigarette smoke caused cancer, but extract of hamburger did not. After many fractionations he found CLA that conferred the protection against cancer.

Fruits and veggies contain cancer fitting phytochemicals[7]. Both black and green tea contains anticarcinogens. These chemicals are particularly effective against lung, colon and skin cancers. These chemicals include catechins, flavins and red color of black tea, all are antioxidants. Also other components in black tea may have antimutagenic effects. The

CANCER CURE via DNA

flavins in tea suppress cancer cell growth in animals at early and late stages of development.

Soybeans contain a group of phytocheminicals called isoflavones, they are found in soybeans. The major isoflavones are daiozein and genistein. These isoflavones may reduce the risk of cancer in many organs..

Blueberries contain anthocyanins, this is the pigment of blueeberries. These anthocyanins may prevent cancer. Proanthocyanidin also found in blueberries inhibit the enzyme involved in the promotion stage of cancer.

These discussed chemicals are antioxidants, as such they neutralize cancer causing chemicals, and they may also neutralize the attachment sites on viruses or attachment sites on the cell from viral attachment, and injection of viral RNA or DNA into the cell.

Processed tomato products may reduce the risk for developing prostate, digestive track and other cancers [36]. Lycopene, a carotenoid, that gives tomatoes their color is a powerful antioxidant. Lycopene has been touted to prevent prostate cancer. Vitamin C, E, and carotene may protect against cancer [6].

Nutritionist say eat at least five servings of fruits and vegetables every day. This regime provides Vitamin C, Vitamin E, and carotenoids. These chemicals play a crucial roles in preventing or delaying cancer. It is thought that these chemicals act as antioxidants. As stated before, Bruce Ames the developer of the Ames test for mutation of microbes, as discussed previously had some interesting observation. He stated that DNA in each cell of human body receives many oxidative insults per day. Most are repaired by the body, but some are not repaired.

Since cancer cases increase significantly in older individuals, it is almost like nature does not care about us once we have reproduced. Oxidative processes are involved in both the initiation of carcinogenesis and the promotion of tumor development.

Antioxidants can be lowered in blood by smoking, illnesses, and other stresses.

Low fat diet may lower the risk of recurrence of breast cancer [21]. Fat increases estrogen production, and estrogen fuels breast cancer or estrogen receptive tumors. Low fat diet only benefits estrogen receptor negative group. There are apparently other mechanisms that play a role in breast cancer.

Linus Pauling discovered Vitamin C [14]. His subsequent work showed that Vitamin C is needed to form interferon, and activate lymphocytes. Lymphocytes destroy viruses and bacteria. In cancer prevention , Dr. Pauling estimates that we need megadoses or 15 grams per day for 150 pound man . Humans still produce the precursor for Vitamin C but we lost the enzyme to convert the precursor to Vitamin C.

At high levels and on a continuous bases Vitamin C can prevent cancer not completely, but significantly. These studies were done with overwhelming amounts of leukemia virus. The suspicion is, that if reasonable amount of viral particles were used, the results would have been even better.

Sunlight and U.V. light cause certain types of skin cancer [27]. The hypothesis is that photochemical conversion of skin cholesterol to carcinogenic substances may play a role in the induction of cancer. Antioxidants like Vitamin C and E may play a role in preventing cancer.

As we discussed previously, U.V. and therefore, sunlight can cause the production of carcinogens, but direct affect on DNA of skin cells is also possible. We do have DNA repair enzymes in our cells, and these enzymes are very affective. But in some of us the enzyme due to U.V. hits on the DNA that produces the enzyme is modified somewhat or more. The enzyme in those individuals may not function properly or not at all. This may explain why some individuals are highly susceptible to skin cancer, while others are not, and everything in between.

It also should be noted, that the carcinogens produced by sunlight and U.V. can react with DNA randomly. If the protein for suppression of a cancer virus is changed, the virus will reproduce and form viruses. If it itself was affected by sunlight or its genes so that production of viruses is not possible, the virus can cause cancer. If the genes that are needed to produce cancer are also damaged – nothing happens. The cell lives until apoptosis takes place.

Chapter 7 References

1. T. James Anderson, Primary Bone Sarcomas of the Dog and Cat, Waltham focus, Vol.6, No. 3, p 21.
2. J. C. Arcos, Cancer: Chemical Factors in the Environment, American laboratory, June 1978, p.29
3. David Baltimore, Viruses, Polymerases, and Cancer, Science, May 14, 1976, p. 632.
4. E. P. Benditt, The Origin of Atherosclerosis, N. Engl. J. Med., Aug. 12, 1976.
5. No Name, Biochemical Markers: Early Warning Sighs of Cancer, Science Vol. 197, Aug., 1977, p. 549.
6. Gladys Black and Lillian Langseth, Antioxidant Vitamins and Disease Prevention, Food Technology, July, 1994, p. 80.

7. Kitty Broihier, Fitting Cancer With Phytochemicals, Food Processing, Nov. 1997, p. 41.
8. John Cairns, The Cancer Problem, Scientific American, Vol. 233, No. 5, Nov. 1975, p. 64.
9. No author, The Great Cancer Virus Race, Laboratory Management, April 1972, p. 16, 18 and 21.
10. Jack Challem, Coenzyme Q 10, The Nutrition Reporter, Oct. 17, 2002.
11. Gepffrey M. Cooper, Cellular Transforming Genes, Science, Vol. 27, 1982, p 801.
12. Max D. Cooper and Alexander R. Lawton III, The Development of the Immune System, Sci. Am., 1974: 231, [5], p 59.
13. C. M. Crole and Hilary Koprowski, The Genetics of Human Cancer, Int. J. Cancer, July 15, 1986, 38 [1], p. 47.
14. More Evidence that Vitamin C Destroys Viruses, Medical World News, Feb. 2, 1977.
15. B.J. Culliton, Cancer Virus Theories: Focus of Research Debate, Science, Vol. 177, July 7, 1972,p. 44.
16. Current Topics, Tumor Virus Program Stirs Controversy and Nostalgia, ASM News, Vol. 58, No.3, 1992, p.126.
17. Matthew C. Dodd, Transferring Cancer Immunity From Animals to human Cells, Science News, Vol. 101, May 27, 1972, p. 341.
18. Renato Dulbecco, From the Molecular Biology of Oncogenic DNA Viruses to Cancer, Science, 92 [4238], April 30, 1976, p. 437.
19. J. Falkman, The Vascularization of Tumors, Sci. Am. May, 1976, 234[5], p. 58.
20. D. Gillespie and R.C. Gallo, RNA Processing and RNA Tumor Virus Origin and Evolution, Science, Vol 188, May 23, 1975, p.802.

21. Health and Wellness, Diet Seen Cutting Recurrence of Breast Cancers, Food Business News, may 24, 2005, p. 24.
22. John E. Illingworth, UV initiation of Cancer, American laboratory, June, 1976, p. 56.
23. Harry L. Ioachim, passive Immunity Achieved Against Leukemia, laboratory management, June, 1972, p. 26.
24. Gina Bari Kolate, Chemical Carcinogens: Industry Adopts Contravertial " Quick" Tests, Science, Vol. 192, June 18, 1976,p. 1215.
25. Ronald Kotulak, Chicago Tribune, Cancer Vaccine, Science Hopeful, Sunday April 1, 1979.
26. Evelyn Leigh, Grape Seed Extract Applications Expand, Prepared Foods, Feb. 2003.
27. Wan- Bang Lo, Homer S. Black, Inhibition of Carcinogen Formation in Skin irradiated with Ultraviolet Light, Nature, Vol. 246, Dec. 21/28, !973, p. 489.
28. Jean L. Marx, Autoimmune Disease, New Evidence About Lupus, Science, Vol. 192, June 11, 1976, p. 1089.
29. Thomas H. Maugh II, The Artificial Gene: it's Synthesis and it's Works in Cell, Science, Vol. 194, Oct., 1976.
30. R. A. Passwater, Cancer New Directions, American Laboratory, June, 1973.
31. H. Graham Purchase, Top Award Goes to Cancer Research, ASM News, Vol. 38, No. 6,June, 1972, p. 309.
32. Reed, is Cancer Man's Middle Name, Science News, Vol. 102, June 29, 1972, p.68.
33. Orlando Sentinel, Sunday, June 15, 2008.
34. R. F. Spark, Legislating Against Cancer, The New Republic, June 3, 1978, p.16.

35. Howard M. Temin, The Relationship of Tumor Virology to an Understanding of Non Viral Cancers, Bio Science, Vol. 27, No.3, March 1977, p. 170.
36. No name, Tomato Products Reduce Cancer Risk, Food Formulating, April 1997, p. 12.
37. Jeanne Turner, Conjugated Linoleic Acid, Food Product Design, Oct. 2003.
38. N. Tsuchida, M. S. Robin and M. Green, Viral RNA subunits in Cells Transformed by RNA Tumor Viruses, Science, Vol. 176, June 30, 1972, p. 1418.
39. Roberts R. Wagner, The 1975 Nobel laureates in Physiology or Medicine, David Baltimore, Renato Dulbeco and Howard Martin Temin.
40. T.D. Waters, Yellow Fever Vaccination, Avian Flu Leukosis Virus, and Cancer Risk in Man, Science, Vol.177, June 7, 1072.
41. Carrie E. Whitmire, Inhibition of chemical Carcinogenesis by Viral Vaccines, Science, Vol. 177, July 7, 1972, p.60

CHAPTER 8
HOW TO CURE CANCER
- A PROPOSAL

HERE ALSO IT IS not so important to understand the complexities that DNA can get into, but only to appreciate the fact that it is complex.

First, the various procedures and treatments are reviewed. Next, indicate that cancer by these treatments is still in most cases not cured. And the one's that appear to be cured, in most likelihood is due to the immune system being mobilized against the specific cancer. To assume anything else is to assume that in the cases were cure is produced, all the cancer cells are eliminated from the body. That assumption is an impossibility.

The author believes strongly in antioxidants, especially if they come from plants or plant extracts. Monkeys that are starved for fruit, develop cancer. Antioxidants are also reviewed in this chapter. This chapter culminates in the proposed cure for cancer, not a cure but a proposal how to cure cancer. Again, this is not been proven yet, but if one followed this book from the beginning to the end, the proposal is the inescapable conclusion.

Can genes predict cancer? This article indicates that you can test for more than 1,500 diseases by looking at the specific genes including cancer of the DNA of these cells [10]. Most of these tests are based on single genes that have mutated. The gene mutation produces a different end product that the original gene. But, these tests at best predict only a 50/50 potential for getting that specific cancer. These are apparently much more in the DNA that is required for a specific cancer. We addressed the cancer virus theories, and showed cancer virus causing cancers in animals. In humans, we do show that viruses isolated from human cancer cells do cause cancers in animals. Some of these human viruses are similar to viruses that cause cancer in animals. Infecting humans with cancer viruses like with animals is not allowed, at least in the U.S. and other civilized countries.

The proposed procedure elaborated later in this chapter in how to cure cancer should be acceptable to the authorities. Note, this is a proposal, it will have to be developed and tested. But, since there are no cures for cancer other than extending life, as indicated in previous chapters, this proposal should be evaluated as soon as possible. As also indicated before, there are exceptions, but as a rule there are no cures to date.

The proposal is based on viruses causing cancer. We did see that carcinogens produce different results than when viruses are used to cause cancer. But, even these results do not preclude the fact that particular cancer produced by carcinogens is not caused by latent virus. In the proposal later, we will be dealing with expressed genes in a cancer. Weather it is viral induced or chemically induced, the cancer cell has to be expressing specific genes that it needs to become cancerous. And, it is many genes not one or two.

Stanley and Cohen used restriction endonucleases to produce so called fragments of a plasmid and then to create a plasmid that once introduced functions as a plasmid [7]. The sticky ends created by endonucleases are zipped up by DNA ligase.

Today it is known that most if not all endonucleases cleave genes apart. Between genes, there are DNA sequences that the endonucleases split and create sticky ends for rejoining. In this situation they produce genes from the plasmid. These genes were separated by gel electrophoreses. The genes are cut out and solubilized. Utilizing DNA ligase one can put together any combination one likes with genes from two dissimilar plasmids. They used transformation to introduce these finished plasmids into E. coli. These procedures could be investigated as a means of incorporating cancer genes into plasmids. These plasmids then can be introduced into selected bacteria.

Nester's book list the known cancer viruses of animal and man [25]. The RNA viruses include arboviruses, myxoviruses, paramyxoviruses, picarnoviruses, reoviruses and rhabdoviruses. The DNA viruses include adenoviruses, herpesviruses, papovaviruses, parvoviruses and poxviruses.

Arboviruses multiply in insects and are transmitted by the insect by injecting the virus into the blood stream of man or animals. There are 200 or more arbovirus.

Myxoviruses causes influenza in man. It has the ability to change with respect to immunity, Different strains seem to appear early, some are more virulent then others.

Paramyxoviruses produce measles and mumps. Today we have vaccines for measles and mumps.

Picarnoviruses includes polioviuses that cause poliomyelitis, coxsackievirus caused intestinal disorders, echovirused cause respiratory to central nervous system infections.

Reoviruses contain double stranded RNA, causes mild respiratory infection to fatal pneumonia, and can cause rashes.

Rhabodoviruses cause rabies in man and some other animals.

Adenoviruses causes respiratory infections.

Herpesviruses is known as cold sore virus, chickenpox and causes shingles.

Papovaviruses cause warts in man.

Poxviruses cause small pox, cow pox and other skin infections.

All of these viruses have been shown to cause cancers in animals. Isolets from humans have been shown to cause cancer in animals. As indicated before, all viral infections do not destroy all cell, but some becomes part of the cell DNA. Under the right conditions the virus can express itself by producing viruses or cause cancer.

There are also viruses that are what is called slow virus. They cause destruction of nerve cells, and the destruction of the myelin sheath. If you loose too many nerve cells, your body does not function properly. If you destroy the myelin sheath, you loose nerve function, the signal does not reach the intended target and gets lost along the way. Ultimately man gets multiple sclerosis. The reason that it is suspected that these diseases are cause by slow viruses , is that these viruses contain RNA – dependent DNA polymerase, which is found in oncogenic viruses.

The immunizing agents that are available for treatment will be stated below, since the final step in the proposed cancer treatment may include one or more of these procedures. Diphtheria and tetanus toxins are prepared for injection into humans by treating the exotoxins by formalin. Many others are killed suspensions of the microbe that causes the specific disease. In Mycobacterium tuberculosis, avirulent strain was discovered and used as a live suspension. Many of the viral vaccines are either used as live virus, formalin killed, or attenuated by growing in animal tissue or in chicken eggs.

McCance treatise on human tumor viruses is in depth analysis of knowledge up to 1998 [19], This book discuses in much more details the tumor viruses than I have done in my book. My intent was to use the data available to indicate that human cancer viruses infection is no different than the bacteriophages infecting bacteria. The human infection may be more complicated than bacterial infections, but still caused by DNA or RNA viruses and therefore, infection of DNA of the individual or its mitochondria in the cells that are transformed into cancer cells.

As stated above the actual immunizing agents are given live or attenuated by variety of procedures including formalin, as will be discussed later. In the case of the bacteria containing the cancer genes, live vaccine may be best. But, attenuated forms should also be tried

What bacteria to use? In my opinion, Bacilus subtilis is the best candidate for cloned gene products, like cancer genes [27].

1. Does not produce disease or toxins.
2. Grows on simple media
3. Since this microbe has been used extensively, much is known how to propagate.

4. Much is known about it's protein membrane permeability should be easily adoptable to excreting foreign proteins.
5. Foreign genes have been introduced and expressed by this bacteria
6. Asporogenous mutants exist, since sporulation terminates cell metabolism.
7. This microbe has been genetically engineered many times
8. No toxicity of any nature resulting from the variety of genetic permutations done with this organism.

One could use other bacteria, fungi, yeast [asporagenous fungi] and mammalian cells or actinomycetes. Unfortunately other bacteria can produce toxins or be pathogenic. Fungi and yeast are eukaryotic and the DNA is complex and hard to deal with. Mammalian cells can bring in new cancer viruses that may complicate the job. Actinomycetes are bacteria like but have many complications, since the gene transfer methods/ systems are still being developed.

Many products that we consume as humans are made by using microbes. Many milk derived products are made by bacteria, like Streptococci, Lactobacilli, Leuconostoc and molds. Wine is made by varieties of Saccharomyces cerevisiae that is a yeast. Beer is also made by Saccharomyces species. Bread is also made using Saccharomyces species. Vinegar is produced by a bacteria called Acerobacter aceti. Sauerkraut is produced by fermentation with bacteria.

Smallpox does not exist as a disease in the world, it is the worst disease that man ever encountered so far [3].

Variolation was first started by the Chinese. Variolation is inhaling the dried crust from a pustule from a afflicted person with small pox. In the east, the dried liquid from small pox sore was scratched into the skin.

Edward Jenner introduced in 1796 the cow pox vaccination for small pox in England, and cow pox later became the vaccine of choice. It is prepared from the dried up sore of cow with cow pox. It was also known that if a person had cowpox, that person then did not get small pox. Cowpox in humans is relatively mild form of pox. Today, the vaccine is prepared from a cross bread virus of cowpox and small pox.

Today, the last small pox incident took place in 1978, since then no small pox incidence anyplace in the world. Small pox has been eradicated according to WHO.

It is interesting to note, that the cow pox pustule produces a liquid, when dried can be used to immunize a person that does not have this dreaded disease. The dried pustule material must be inactive virus, otherwise, you would produce the disease. The body produces antibodies against the dead component of the inactive virus. In the case of cow pox the infection is not as severe as small pox and afterword the person is protected against small pox. It obviously has gene products that are similar to small pox, but does not have the genes to cause as severe infection as small pox. It's dried up liquid from the pustule also protects. This is similar situation in terms of protection as T.B. vs. T.B. of cows.

The cross bread virus of cow pox and small pox is being used to prepare vaccines against other viruses, like rabies, aids, hepatitis B, influenza, herpes simplex and many other viruses. All these preparations are developed by introducing into the virus genes of the other viruses to produce antibodies against their end products dictated by their specific genes. To date, we have not found any new viruses produced in a individual or animal due to the virus in the individual or animal reacting with the cow pox/small pox virus and creating a new even more potent virus.

The virus also should be considered for the later proposed immunization/cure of cancer viruses. In the cure situation, the identified cancer genes should be put into the cow pox/small pox virus to determine if the genes products of the cancer virus when expressed will cause the bodies immune system to recognize these being non self and attack them as well as the cancer. Also, if you know for sure that a specific virus in an individual will cause cancer. Put the genes of that virus into the cow pox/small pox virus and try to immunize that individual long before the cancer would have developed.

It also may not be to far fetched to follow the above example by causing human cancer in susceptible animals, taking the cancerous tissue, grinding it up, and drying, and then scratching the dried tissue into the skin of that individual with that cancer. This may be a way of causing the body to recognize non self in the tissue, and once these non self components are recognized, the body attacks the cancer.

Louis Pasteur was a microbiologist par excellence, He worked on the chemistry of fermentation, diseases of wine and beer, destroyed spontaneous generation, worked on silk worm disease, immunization against foul cholera, anthrax, swine erysipelas and rabies.

Pasteur developed a method to cultivate the rabies virus in the medulla of rabbits and attenuate the virus by drying fragments of medulla in sterilized vials. Even today 13 inoculations of Pasteur's vaccine over consecutive 10 days , protects the individual from rabies.

These are examples of viruses attenuated by drying and used to cause a immunity response to the specific virus.

Apoptosis is the orderly dying of a cell [37]. Orderly death is build into cells for many reasons. In the immune system the T-cells and the B –cells exhibit orderly death. In T-cells death is invited when the T-cell encounters what it suppose to destroy. B-cells produce antibodies then they die. When a virus like a cancer virus infects a human cell, the cell tries to prevent the viral infection by apoptosis. So, the cell dies before the virus infection establishes itself in the cell. But, the viral DNA or RNA produces inhibitors that prevent apoptosis, and the cell goes into a growth cycle. This only takes place in situations were the virus is a cancer virus that causes cancer or the virus needs the cell to grow so that the virus can replicate its progenies. In a cell were the virus becomes part of the DNA of the cell, the cell does not change its growth characteristics.

Murine sarcoma virus can both transform and replicate in mouse cells in the presence of murine leukemia virus, but can only transform them in it's absence [11].

Cells containing murine sarcoma virus were cultured, colonies that appeared normal were isolated. Subjecting these colonies to murine leukemia virus did not produce murine sarcoma virus. Also these cells do not contain RNA- dependent DNA polymerase. What is going on here? It would appear as we discussed before, these cells are transformed and the virus is integrated and shut off from expressing by the repressor molecule. As we know now, in animals there could be many viruses that have been integrated through generations. Only by subjecting these cells to carcinogens do we release latent viruses. A simpler explanation may be that in the virus the genes have been damaged, and it has no functional RNA-dependent DNA polymerase.

Singer and Garth L Nicolson developed the fluid mosaic model of the cell membrane. The membranous bilayer consist of phospholipids [28]. The water soluble heads are on the outside in the aqueous environment. The tails which are lipid are inside the membrane called lipid bilayer. Proteins stick through the membrane creating chemicals, cell surface antigens, etc.

Most likely, cell mediated immunity or antibody dedicated immunity do not enter the cell, but deal with the surface proteins – antigens.

It is assumed, that cancer cells surface is different then the normal cell surface. But, if that is correct, why does the immune system not recognize the cancer surface as non self and destroy the cancer cells? The question is still not answered. It could be that the cancer cell produces a cloaking mechanism which has to be in the cancer DNA. Taking the cancer genes and transferring them to another living thing or virus and immunizing with other living thing or virus, may uncloak the cancer cell. The cancer is recognized and destroyed.

Drug Avastin blocks the growth of blood vessels [1]. But the drug can cost $92,000/year. The treatment is radiation and drugs and Avastin. It prolongs life but does not cure the disease

Chemicals affecting tumors – Synthetic Cocoa chemicals slow growth of tumors.

Synthetic chemical based on chemicals in cocoa beans slowed growth and accelerated destruction of human tumors in lab tests. This compound is in class of procyanidins which is a class of flavanols [but synthetic not natural]. This patented synthetic chemical was developed by Mars Incorporated. This chemical is especially effective in treating fast growing cancer cells. Do not know how it works, other than maybe it is a powerful antioxidant, it interferes with the cancer cells

As we have stated before, tumor viruses or chemical carcinogens could convert normal cells to transformed cells.

The belief is that transformed cells produce different proteins than normal cells [2]. Therefore, scientists have been looking for proteins that are different from normal cells. They found a protein that appears to prevent cells from growing wildly and not in monolayers. Transformed cells do not have this protein, and there are many other changes in the surface of the cell that protein produce. It would appear that these changes produce the condition called cancer.

In this article, they focus on the large surface protein that is lost when cells are transformed. And, almost gave credence to the fact that the loss of this protein causes cancer. If that is so, then one gene causes cancer. That is hard to believe, as we discussed in previous chapters concerning breast cancer. In breast cancer a single gene is present in cancer patients that is used to predict breast cancer. Very small proportion of people that have this gene succumb to breast cancer.

In my opinion, not a single gene or a single protein causes cancer. It has to be at the very minimum the expression of multiple genes of a latent virus. Both the gene in breast cancer and the large surface protein which is a byproduct of a gene may be involved, but cannot be the cause of cancer by itself.

Glucose infusions into cancer colony causes lactic acid production which lowers the pH [15]. Normal pH is slightly above neutral , which is the normal mean value, it can go down to just above neutral pH. Note: it is not neutral or acidic but slightly basic.

Harguinbey and Gillis believe that lowering the pH to just above neutral can cause the immune system to respond, and in some cases the cancer regresses or disappears. Could it be due to the cancer cell under lower pH conditions goes into

Anthony J Luksas PhD

apoptosis. Cancer cells normally live forever or as long as the subject lives.

Harguindey and Kolbeck concluded that there is still no real understanding of cancer [14].

They indicated, that if respiration is interfered with, that is the cause of cancer or the cell dies. According to the them, that is based on the best available evidence to date.

As previously discussed, the mitochondria is the energy mill and produces ATP's. it has its own DNA. The DNA is bacterial. Is it possible that infection with bacterial viruses transforms the mitochondrial DNA into cancer. Unfortunately, the author is not aware of any research in this area, like comparing mitochondrial DNA of good cell of a specific organ with a cancerous cell mitochondrial DNA from the same organ.

The article addresses the various ways of explaining metastasis [26] . They address the fact that not every cell that splits off the original cancer establishes colonies [metastasis]. The other issue is that metastasis does not take place in all other organs of the body. Breast cancer goes to brain or lungs, lung cancer goes to brain and adrenal glands, prostate cancer to bone.

They found that when a cancer should send out cells to create metastasis, if that animal is challenged with specific microbes, metastasis does not take place. The microbes used were Bacillus Calmette – Guerin [BCG] or Corynebacterium parvum

Apparently, the immune system is stimulated to destroy the cells that produce metastasis. Obviously, the question is, how does this work. They concluded that most likely the immune system recognizes the microbes as non self and produces antibodies against their surface antigens. The bacterial antigens have enough similarity to the cancer cells surface proteins that the immune system recognizes them as non-self and destroys them.

In contrast to normal cells, cancer cells have lost the ability to stop dividing after contact with its neighbor [23]. This is due to cell surface receptors.

There are attempts to discover why some cancer cells escape destruction by host's immune defense system even though their altered surface components betray them as being non self.

As stated before, Singer and Nicolson came up with the cell membrane as fluid-mosaic. The cell membrane is one-half millionth of an inch. It is composed of proteins, phospholipids and sugar polymers. Note that specific plant proteins bind to specific sugar polymers attached to cell membrane. Two specific plant proteins from toxic wild caster plants causes cancer cells to form balls.. There is no effect on normal calls. Even though, normal cell membranes do bind some number of these specific plant proteins.

One specific plant protein when viewed under electron microscope, binds to normal cell in a dispersed fashion, but in tumor cell the specific plant protein binding is bunched up and not dispersed.

Why do some cancer cells escape the immune system? One theory is that the cancer cells are coated with antibodies to a surface proteins that did not destroy the cancer. You need to expose the other proteins to the immune system, at this time there was no knowledge how to it.

One other theory looks at surface molecule arrangement so as to not be recognizes as non self.

The third theory states that the cancer cell when attacked by antibodies or T – cells retract the proteins into the surface membrane.

One or all theories may be true, but at this time these are theories only. What we do know now is that the cancer cell cloaks itself well from the immune system.

Researchers have studied spontaneous regression of cancer [24]. In three cases of melanoma, the patients received blood from patients recovering from melanoma, and their melanomas disappeared. This indicates that in patients that recovered from melanoma, the immune system recognized the cancer cells as non self and destroyed it.

There is no indication how these patients became melanoma free. The only thing that we can say, is that these are visible changes in patients that recovered from melanoma. These changes can be thyroid gland enlargement, infection with bacteria producing high fever, reoccurring malaria.

One patient with breast cancer, and with metastases became a drunk. With the heavy drinking the primary cancer and metastasized cancer disappeared. With no apparent cancer remaining for 10 years subsequent to treatment, but high intake of alcohol. When the patient died at the end of 10 years, coroner indicated high blood alcohol and arrested cancer in bone marrow.

It is important to note, that cancer cells are not foreign like bacteria or viruses, but are native cells of the host that have become cancerous [4]. But, there may be viruses that get into the cell, or latent viruses that become active in those cells. These latent viruses are inherited from parents, grand parents and so forth.

Even when cancer is treated in many cases cancer cells can be detected in the blood stream. And yet, there is no cancer. It is almost like there is immunity present.

The objective of orthomolecular treatment is to enhance natural resistance to cancer to maximum efficiency in every patient. In autopsy, there is a good chance that cancer is found in a arrested state. To enhance natural resistance one should use physiological means. Use nutrients, minerals, trace elements, vitamins and hormones.

Hormones do not directly act against cancer cells, but create unfavorable environment for cancer to proliferate. Vitamins, like vitamin C holds promise, providing the environment is also controlled with other components. Ascorbic acid is involved in many chemical reactions that may create unfavorable environment for cancer.

Good collagen to create dense fibrous tissue to encase cancer colony is needed. Vitamin C is a cofactor to an enzyme that converts proline to hydroxiproline. Hydroxiproline is essential to the formation of good collagen. The human body does not produce hydroxiproline, only proline. Scurvy, is the lack of vitamin C, which leads to two dimensional not three dimensional collagen . Two dimensional collagen forms poor connective tissue. The major effect is bleeding, which is caused by the blood vessels breaking and eventually the person dies. There is also a need to have high concentration of ascorbic acid in adrenal & pituitary glands. Stress depletes the ascorbic acid from these glands, and corresponding decrease in hormone production.

Hyaluronidase is released by neoplastic cells, which helps the cancer to spread. If sufficient amount of vitamin C is in the system, providing other necessary components of orthomolecular medicine are incorporated, the body produces sufficient hyaluronidase inhibitor [PHI]. This enzyme inhibits hyaluronidase and helps prevent cancer from spreading. Sufficient amount of vitamin helps also the immune system to function properly.

Viruses are inactivated by vitamin C. Vitamin C acts on Rous sarcoma virus, herpes virus which causes carcinoma of cervix and Epstein-Barr virus [a herpes virus], that causes Burkett's lymphoma.

Ascorbic acid content of leucocytes influence their phagocytic activity and enhances host resistance to infections. Cameron and Pauling indicated that when experimental animals are challenged with carcinogen that can induce cancer, the animal produces significantly more Vitamin C, of the order of 100 to 200 fold.

Cameron and Campbell article discusses the results of 50 untreatable cancer patients exposed to high levels of Vitamin C [5]. The treatment extended life of terminal cancer patients from 3 – 659 month. At least 5 patients showed regression of cancer, but ultimately they died, except one, that was alive and went to work at the writing of this article. The treatment with Vitamin C was at 10g./day. In all cases there were improvements in norbidity, there was less pain, and other symptoms were reduced significantly.

Death when it comes with Vitamin C, in most of the 50 patients is precipitous and the patient dies in a few days.

Patient No. 45 in previous manuscript. This patient was terminal due to extensive metastasis. Vitamin C at high levels [10g/day] were prescribed and eventually went in complete remission. The cancer came back following Vitamin C removal from treatment due to remission. The Vitamin C at higher levels [i.e. 20g/day for 14 days, then 12.5g/day oraly there after] was started and again complete remission.

The patient continued to take 12.5g/day and has returned to work. At the writing of this article, the patient continued to work.

Cancer patience have a much greater requirement for Vitamin C, than non cancer patients [6]. Vitamin C plays a role in many immune responses to cancer.

In this report they placed 100 terminal patients on 10g/day of Vitamin C, intravenous for 10 days, then 10g/day orally. This was compared to 1,000 patients that were also declared terminal. The 100 and the 1,000 were being helped with cancer treatment. The results indicated 3 – 20 times longer survival on Vitamin C.

Cameron and Pauling indicated as was indicated in the previous references that if treatment with Vitamin C was at higher level, like in the previous article, 20g/day and subsequent 12.5g/day every day until death, the survival would be increased significantly. Also, if treatment with Vitamin C was started earlier in cancer treatment, the survival may be 5 – 20 years.

Antibiotics allowed treatment of bacterial diseases [18]. Discovery of penicillin by Alexander Fleming started the antibiotic era. That started in the mid 1940's and helped save lives in W.W. II. Today these are many different antibiotics, as well as modified penicillins to avoid resistance by bacteria.

The era of antiviral drugs started in the 1970's. unlike antibiotics used to treat bacteria which are completely effective. Sometime one has to use a combination of antibiotics or different antibiotic to kill bacteria, but the outcome is essentially always positive. There are bacterial diseases that can be very hard to cure and at least in one case, the flesh eating bacteria – fatal.

The first approved antiviral medicine was idoxuridine, and was sold as stoxil by Smith Kline & French Laboratory of

Philadelphia. It is effective against herpes keratitis, which causes eye infection that can lead to blindness. It is used externally only. If administered internally, the drug has many side affects. Not used for any other use as a drug.

The second was methisazone, sold as marboran by Burroughs Wellcome Co. It is very effective against small pox and cow pox. Since small pox is gone from the human population on this earth, it is a drug in search of a disease. The next drug was Amantadine hydrochloride sold as symmentetrel by Endo Laboratories. It is affective against influenza. FDA did not approve the drug, so it is not used.

Another drug is riboverin, in herpes infections it interferes with the production of the nucleotides, and therefore, the production of viruses. Ribovirin is also useful against herpes zoster [shingles] as a salve, not for internal use. It is also effective against hepatitis A [an RNA virus}, but not against hepatitis B an DNA virus]. It is also effective against influenza, which is a RNA virus. The drug inhibits production of viral proteins, but does not inhibit host's protein production.

Another anti viral drug is vidarabine [ademome arabinoside, developed by Parks Davis Company of Detroit. It works against pox viruses, oncornaciruses, and rhabdiviruses. It works also very well against herpes viruses. It apparently blocks DNA polymerase of the virus, and prevents viral production. The drug is effective against herpes keratitis.

Another viral drug is phosphonoacetic acid. It is affective against herpes viruses. It also inhibits the viral DNA polymerase

Influenza virus causes epidemic, while most viruses do not, excluding of course small pox. In small pox case it has been eradicated, while influenza virus is not. How is that possible?

It was determined that influenza virus can exchange genes with different viral strains.

If two influenza virus infect a cell, when the two viruses reproduce and undergo rearrangement of their genes and produce one or more viruses that have genes from each. The difference in the new viruses is their glycoprotein. The immune system does not have antibodies to the new glycoprotein. These new viruses can cause another influenza. In the future, and when the body immune system recognizes the new surface glycoprotein and stops the infection, new influenza viruses are created. For whatever reason the new viruses created in the particular body do not re -infect, the body these new viruses are created in.

Influenza B & C do not follow influenza A in rearrangement or exchange of genes, and therefore, do not cause epidemics.

During the Hong Kong influenza of 1968 – 1969 E.I. du Pont requested FDA to use the drug amantadine hydrochloride named synetrel against this variance of influenza. FDA said no, 40,000 people died from this virus in U.S.

E.I. du Pont tested this drug against Asian A2 strain and found a significant effect in reducing the severity of the disease. Which probably would have saved the lives that were lost.

The drug was finally approved for influenza A2, but by then the epidemic was over. When DuPont requested the drug to be used on strains that caused influenza coming from the origin A2 strains, FDA rejected the petition. They finally approved the drug use after Du Pont did extensive trials, but it was too late, the infection subsided.

There was questions raised why FDA rejected the petition. FDA decision was based on the fact that the advisory group that was convened to evaluate the petition rejected the petition. As later it was found, the advisory group had a stake in vaccines used in influenzas.

This act of FDA almost stopped viral drug production. How did it survive? It was found to be very effective against Parkinson's disease. Symetrel was approved by FDA for that use in 1973.

Other countries did evaluate the drug and found the drug to be effective against many influenza variants.

It is interesting to note, that a viral drug works effectively on Parkinson's disease. Is Parkinson's disease viral in origin, is it some form of cancer?

U.S. congress directed in 1955 the National Cancer Institute [NCI] to start Drug development program [12]. This activity still exists at NCI.

The program focus was on leukemias and lymphomas. They tried a combination of chemicals. In early1960's their cure rate was 50 – 60 % in children with leukemia. In Hodgkin's and non Hodgkin's lymphoma there was also cures. With Bleomycin, Cisplatin, and Adriamycin they got 70 – 80 % cure of testicular cancer that was metastasized.

The cures as discussed above were achieved in cancers that did not metastasize. If the tumor metastasized, the cure did not work as well.

These drugs besides attacking tumor cells, also attack growing cells like bone marrow, stomach, and hair follicle.

Most of the chemicals used are themselves carcinogenic. If Hodgkin's disease is treated with these chemicals that are carcinogenic, the chemicals may cure Hodgkin's disease but they may induce leukemia. Other cancers if treated with chemotherapy may also develop other tumors.

In my opinion, these chemotherapeutic chemicals can induce and promote latent cancers. These chemical treatments when they supposedly cause regression, this may be due to the body recognizing the non self cells and starts to destroy them. These chemicals cause cancer cell death. In doing so, they releases various cell components. Some of these cancer cell components differ from normal cell components. If the immune system is not totally inactive due to these chemicals, it reacts and causes regression.

For colorectal cancer need high fiber, fast throughput – less time to develop cancer chemicals [21]. Fast throughput does not allow these cancer chemicals to cause cancer, it has low residence. High intake of fruits and /or vegetable protects against many cancers.

Broccoli, tomatoes and garlic are good against cancer. Broccoli and other cruciferous vegetables contain antioxidants, these have anti cancer activity

Tomatoes and other vegetables & fruits contain lycopene, which is an antioxidant and protects against prostate cancer. Garlic and onions lower the risk of prostate and other cancers.

Asians eat a lot of soy products, they have low incidents of breast and prostate cancer. Dairy products may help in intestinal cancer prevention due to calcium and vitamin D.

As stated before, Asians that consumed soy sauce had high incidence of stomach cancer. Today that cancer is same as other countries or lower. That is due to soy sauce produced in plants that control the microbes used in grain preparation for fermentations.

Also, all the antioxidants found in vegetables, fruit, and various grains are cancer preventers. Since cancer appears to be due to inherited or acquired cancer causing viruses, the antioxidants act on the attachment of viruses to cells as well as preventing damage to DNA.

The specific antioxidants associated with specific cancer prevention are derived from population studies. Example, Italians eat a lot of tomatoes, tomatoes have the antioxidant lycopene. Italians have a low incidence of prostate cancer. Therefore, lycopene protects against prostate cancer. Unfortunately, an association does not prove cause and affect. But, this is so ingrained in literature, it now is assumed as fact.

American Institute for Cancer Research [AICR] and the World Health Organization recommends food intake to consist of large amounts of fruits and vegetables and low amounts of meat and moderate amount of alcoholic drinks [20]. They consider fish as meat. Also physical activity is a must as well as weight control.

Antioxidants scavenge free radicals and which if not neutralized can interact with DNA and cause cancer. Carcinogens are free radicals. Vitamins like Vitamin A, beta- carotine, Vitamin C, and Vitamin E are antioxidants and prevents cancer by reacting with free radicals and neutralizing their action.

Vitamin E acts on the markers for cancer, developed or to develop. It is assumed that by lowering the amount of markers on the prostate cell, that may prevent expression of genes that cause cancer. In laboratory experiments, Vitamin E inhibits growth of prostate cancer cells. In addition Vitamin D and selenium are suspect in prostate cancer prevention.

Lycopene and prostate cancer were covered in previous reference as well as selenium. If selenium was not a element it would be a Vitamin, since it is needed for the enzyme glutathione peroxidase. This enzyme detoxifies peroxides that are formed in animals and man,

Grape skin extract contains resveratrol which is an antioxidant. It was shown that resveratrol acts on initiation, promotion, and progression of cancer. This was substantiated utilizing animals and human cells and human cancer cells.

A researcher at U.S. Dept. of Agriculture's Agricultural Research Service [ARS] isolated another compound from grapes that has similar affect on cancer as resveratrol.

In green tea, there are flavonoids which are antioxidants. It was found that green tea is more powerful than Vitamin C or Vitamin E in preventing cancer. These conclusions are based on animal studies.

In broccoli sulforaphane a isothiocyanate is a direct antioxidant that attacks free radicals were they can react with DNA and cause cancer. Antioxidants become active from cooking, physical disruption of the tissue, or mastacation.

Phytochemicals are in soybeans. There is evidence that soybeans prevent cancer. Isoflavone is a phytochemical and is suspected to protect against cancer. Research with isoflavone extract in lab. cultures of cancer cells were shown to inhibit cancer cell growth.

Calcium is suspected to have a positive affect on colon cancer. Vitamin D also is a suspect as having positive affect on colon cancer.

DNA damage is caused by free radicals, produced continuously in our cells, taken in as food or by inhalation. Therefore, cells are continuously becoming damaged and cancerous, but these cells are eliminated by cell death called apoptosis.

But some cells when it's DNA is damaged do not die, but proliferate and become cancer. Anti inflammatory drugs and antioxidants are suspect in preventing these cells from becoming cancerous.

The discovery of P-53 gene put this dilemma into focus, this gene regulates apoptosis. If the cells DNA becomes damaged, the P-53 gene prevents cell division until DNA damage is repaired. But, if repair is not possible it starts apoptosis by starting the process of cell death. If the P-53 gene in DNA is itself damaged by free radicals, and it no longer functions, the damaged cells genetically can become cancer.

Gene therapy is replacing or adding genes, to replace genes that were mutated, or cause the production of specific proteins that relates to cancer so as to cause the immune system to react and destroy the cancer [13]. Gene therapy has the potential of helping to cure cancer. In degenerative diseases the non functional single gene replacement would be possible and functional. They use viruses to infect and deposit the needed gene. One problem with viral inserting a new gene is the problem of the production of inhibitor protein that prevents the expression of the specific gene without the whole virus developing new viruses.

They tried to strip the surface proteins from cancer cells and cause antibody production in the patient with cancer. The results were encouraging but the cancer was not eliminated. They concluded that the body did not produce enough antibodies. Two other possibilities, one , not all the proteins were removed for antibody production, the other, the cancer cell mutated and became resistant to the treatment. As will be discussed later, we should be starting with DNA of the cancer cell, and not the products of the DNA of the cancer cell.

This approach in treating cancer is not likely to succeed. In cancer, every cell that is cancerous has to be destroyed. There is no way to assure that the virus or free DNA as plasmid will reach and infect every cancer cell. Those cancer cells not infected will continue to multiply and continue the cancer.

As in the previous article, the results were the same, not all the cancer cells were destroyed.

Shin article describes producing antibodies against cancer cells, by attenuating the cancer cells, and injecting the cancer cells into mice [36]. After some interval of time antibodies were produced from the immunized cells.

Other mice were inoculated with live cancer cells, to produce solid tumor as well as growing tumor cells in the animal. The antibodies were used to destroy the growing tumor cells as well as the solid tumor. Tumors were not completely suppressed. They concluded that there are more tumor cells then antibodies. Another possibility, they described, was the finding that cancer cells released a factor or factors that interfered with the antibodies.

Also, they concluded that if these mice were first treated with anti cancer drugs, that would reduce the number of cancer cells in the mouse, would treatment with antibodies work. That was not done at this time.

Again, as this article indicates, if they produced antibodies against products of the cancer DNA and not just surface antigens, would that work. The proposal at the end of this chapter addresses that very issue.

There seems to be in animals an immune surveillance for cancer cells [16]. In animals and man tumor cells are continuously produced, but the immune surveillance system determines that these cells are non self and destroys them. But, therefore, when tumors develop, they escape the immune surveillance system. The assumption is that when the immune surveillance system is ineffective, cancer develops. But, cancer develops also in so called individuals with no known immune deficiency. They introduced the blocking factors, that is lumps of antigen and antibody produces a blocking factors where lymphocytes cannot attack the cancer cells. We discussed the immune system before. T-cells produce lymphocytes, and B –cells produce antibodies. Another possibility is that the cancer cell produces antigens that can attach to the lymphocytes and prevent them from attacking the cancer cell. Something like it produces free antigen [s] and the same antigen is in the membrane of the cell. The free antigen neutralizes the lymphocytes. And also, it is possible that tumors do not elicit strong immune response, and therefore, tumors grow while other cancer cells that do elicit strong response do not. They brought into the area of immunity macrophages, these cells have to recognize the cancer cell as foreign, then they engulf and digest the cancer cell.

Bacillus Calmette – Guerin [BCG] is a reduced infectivity strain of bovine tuberculosis [17]. It is used as vaccine against human tuberculosis. Humans can get bovine tuberculosis, but this strain can protect against bovine tuberculosis and human tuberculosis. BCG has been used against cancer. Treatment with BCG can be dangerous, it usually has secondary affects that can be from uncomfortable to death.

When it works it is suspected to induce the immune response to the cancer. The reaction by the immune response may be due to activation of macrophages. The tumor cells are digested within the macrophages and releases tumor antigens that then elicit the immune response to the tumor cells.

Another approach is to attenuate the cancer cells or use tumor surface antigens to cause a immune response.

Normal and cancer cells have sialic acid on the outside of the cell. There is more sialic acid on cancer cells than normal cells; and ,this may be the reason why the immune system does not react to cancer. Therefore, producing via DNA the antigens in a different organism like bacteria may be the answer.

It is interesting to note, that immunotherapy no matter if using BCG, whole cancer cells, cancer cell antigens or new raminidase [enzyme that removes sialic acid] did not eliminate the cancer, it reduced, but did not destroy the cancer.

It is important to note, that using whole cancer cells or the surface proteins can cause the immune system destruction of good cells. This can happen, if the cancer cell contains also normal surface antigens found in normal surface antigens found in normal cells. Better to use only antigens specific to cancer. This is done by taking only cancer genes, transferring these to a bacteria, and treating the individual with the bacteria containing the antigens produced by the bacteria from the cancer genes.

Bacteria can transfer genes to other bacteria, we discussed this in one of the previous chapters. We also discussed bacterial genes transfer into human cells [22].

Bacteria that can invade animal or human cells are absorbed by the cells outer membrane forming a vacual. Once on the cell the bacteria lyse and release their DNA inside the cell, the DNA ends up in the nucleus. Once in the nucleus the bacterial genes can express.

This is useful to treat cancer, and other diseases.

1st, this is clear indication that not only virus but also bacteria can and do transfer genetic material to the mammalian host cells. This like viral DNA can exist in the mammalian cell[s] through generations or be acquired from the environment. As such, they can be involved in producing cancer.

2nd, This approach in curing cancer, unless something unusual happens in the future, cannot cure cancer completely. Every cancer cell has to be infected for cure to tale place. Since, as the article indicates, this process has cured some mice. Most likely, the perturbation of the cancer by these bacterial cells, can cause the infected cells to release its content into the body. These components do circulate in the blood steam and immune system picks the various products and starts to produce antibodies and then destroy all the cancer cells and not just cells that were infected by viruses or absorbed DNA from the environment.

But, this approach is still not good enough. The various methods used today like chemotherapy and radiation can also cause the bodies defense mechanisms to recognize components in dying cells and produce antibodies. There is a better way, which will be discussed later.

Lung cancer is the No.1 killer in women, followed by cancer of the breast [35]. In all cancers especially breast, cancer early detection is very important for survival. In the last 30 + years, drugs have been developed that attack specific molecules on the surface of the tumors. It is interesting to note that men decreased cigarette smoking, while women increased about 20 – 30 years ago. Cancer develops after the specific gene[s] are changed, and it takes about 20 – 30 years for cancer to develop. Breast cancer is a solid tumor cancer.

In 1998 Trastuzumab [herceptin] a drug against breast cancer was approved This drug attacks Her 2. Her 2 promotes aggressive tumor growth . It is important to note, that breast cancer is not a single disease.

It was discovered that BRCA1 gene can increase the risk for cancer significantly. BRCA1 is involved in DNA repair. DNA and therefore, genes are bombarded with carcinogens, U.V., etc. that cause single and double breaks in DNA. If the repair mechanism is faulty other genes can be mutated.

Majority of breast cancers are dependent for survival and growth on estrogen or progesterone. The cancer cells have receptor proteins in the cell membrane for these hormones.

Tamoxifen was approved to treat breast cancer in 1977.The drug attaches to the estrogen or progesterone sites and therefore, prevents the hormones from binding to these sites. Newer drugs have superceded tamoxifen like herceptin.

Sex hormones cause normal cells to grow and multiply and so do cancer cells. Newer knowledge indicates that these are genes that cause normal cells to become cancerous. These genes are called oncogenes. This is not surprising, almost axiomatic, since all normal and cancerous cells are controlled by DNA and therefore, genes.

Breast cancer is not one cancer, but many. Therefore, it will take many drugs to cure these cancers. Approaching the many cancers by developing drugs for each will take years if not forever. Other drugs are being developed to target HER2. Sex hormones cause the proliferation of breast and prostate cancers.

A drug was developed that prevents blood vessel formation to and into tumors. Tumors do not grow in size by cell multiplication without food which has to be supplied to the cancer cells just like healthy cells by blood vessels. If one can inhibit the formation of blood vessels in the tumor, the tumor stops growing and can potentially apoptosize.

Unfortunately the drug does not prevent growth of vessels completely.

Another drug that is a dual EGER/HER2 inhibitor that has shown remarkable laboratory results. This drug leads to cell apoptosis in breast cancer cell lines that over produceHER2.

A alternative means of interfering with cancer growth is importan because, cancer cells often do eventually find ways to evade individual drugs.

By the way, 80% of breast tumors do not have HER2 mutations.

In 70 and 80's some physicians had patients that had lymphomas [34]. The lymphomas decreased but did not completely disappear after they had measles. This led in the 1990's to creating viruses that specifically kills cancer cells. Initially and now they use the common cold virus to create viruses that specifically enter cancer cells and by causing the virus to reproduce within the cancer cell and kill the cancer cell.

Other viruses as cancer killers have also been tried. To date these modified viruses also have the potential of killing normal cells.

Using viruses after modification to kill cancer cells is dangerous and has questionable effectiveness. The author is questioning if this approach will kill all the cancer cells. If the virus does not kill all cancer cells, the cancer will reappear and usually with vengeance. The only way to kill every cancer cell is to cause the immunity in the individual to recognize the cancer cell as non self and destroy every cancer cell.

By the way, It is hard to believe that attaching a promoter gene to a virus will cause the virus to come off the DNA and replicate. The cancer genes are functioning in cancer, if one could cause the virus whose genes are expressed, and that causes the cell to become cancerous, that would indicate that the virus has lost the ability to replicate and therefore the outcome is cancer. As discussed before, there may be numerous viruses that were inherited or acquired during the beings existence. By assuming that the viral therapy causes the specific virus genes causing the cancer to acquire the ability to reproduce, it is more likely the treatment may cause other latent viruses to come off and destroy the cancer cell. That may be OK with respect to killing the specific cancer cell; but, one has to ask, what these newly released viruses doing in the individual.

Porphyria is a disease caused by the depositing of porphyrins in the skin[38]. Some of the porphyrins are transformed by light into skin destroying toxins. Disfiguration of the skin and other organs can take place. But the key is that cells like skin cells take up the porphyrins and then get killed by exposure to light. Many biological polymers in life contain pophyrins, chlorophyll, hemoglobin and many enzymes. Chemicals in garlic interact with light to make the disease more pronounced.

Many diseases of the skin are treated with porphyrins, and other light sensitive chemicals, like psoralens from seeds. It appears that these chemicals when activated by light react with DNA in growing cells and the cell dies.

The idea of using these chemicals or synthetic ones to treat cancer cells started in 70's. porphyrins accumulate in cancer cells since cancer cells are growing cells, and light can therefore activate the porphyrins and kill the cancer cells. Unfortunately, one cannot depend on this to destroy all cancer cells.

The reason that porphyrins accumulate in some people is because the feedback inhibition does not work in some people for these compounds. The excess is deposited in the skin.

Jain in his studies found that abnormal blood vessels are part of cancer [33]. The abnormality is severe and grotesque. They found that anticancer drugs were not delivered effectively to the cancer cells. The delivery was uneven or not at all.

They found that drugs that were designed to destroy blood vessels, did in fact destroy some, but repaired others. That provided on opportunity to deliver anticancer drugs due to some vessels being normalized. Unfortunately, this normalization does not last. The cancer continues producing growth factors to cause new blood vessels to develop. But, there exist a window of opportunity to deliver drugs during the period when the blood vessels are normalized. It is interesting to note, that methods were developed of tracking certain molecules within blood vessels and tissue. It is also interesting to note, that they developed methods of visualizing genes turning on and turning off.

The reason that blood vessels develop abnormally is due to overproduction of growth factors and under production of inhibitory factors. When a wound heals, the growth factors exceed the inhibitory factors. When it is healed, the growth factors are neutralized by inhibitory factors. That does not happen in cancer, and that is why the blood vessels are so grotesque.

Drugs were developed to treat the production of growth factors in many ways, but unfortunately the cancer cells eventually find other ways to produce abnormal vessels. The good news is, that the research succeeded in extending the normal vessels for up to 28 days.

One of the drugs used for normalization is recentin, and as long as the drug is taken, normalization persists. If the drug is removed, the blood vessels become abnormal. The reason the drug is removed, is due to the drugs side affects. When the drug is reintroduced, normal blood vessels are the result.

The newer knowledge of the immune system came into view in 1994 [32]. White blood cells called monocytes give rise to dendritic cells or macrophages. Dendritic cells control the immune system. Macrophages travel throughout the body destroying dead cells and viruses, bacteria, yeast and molds.

Dendritic cells engulf foreign objects, take them apart, and extrude the pieces [antigens] onto their surface. Then they get into either the blood or lymph nodes and end up in the spleen. The surface antigens are recognized by the T-cells. The T-cells educate the B-cells, which produce antibodies against the antigens on the surface of the dendritic cells. The dendritic cells also get the killer T-cells to destroy cells that contain viruses.

It is assumed that cancer cells contain surface antigens that differ from normal cell antigens. In this scenario, the dendritic cells display cancer antigens as well as normal cell antigens. If the immune system makes a mistake and produces antibodies against the normal cell antigens, we end up with lupus, diabetes, or rheumatoid arthritis.

Therefore, lupus and other degenerative diseases occur without treatment for cancer via the dendritic cells. It is important that only the cancer antigens attach to dendritic cells, and only antibodies and killer T-cells are produced against the cancer antigens only. The proposal at the end of this chapter takes that into consideration.

How does inflammation aid cancer? When cytokins also known as tumor necrosis factor [TNF] are injected directly into a cancer colony [31], it kills cancer cells. But, if TNF at a low level exists in cancer, the cancer survives. But, if TNF is shut off, the mice in the experiment did not develop a tumor, that is, the genes producing cytokine was destroyed.

Inflammation can either help cancer or become an obstacle. In most cases the damaged genes start cancer, but inflammation causes the cancer to grow.

As we discussed before, cancer has three stages, initiation, may last for 20 – 30 years; promotion appears to require inflammation to start; progression is when cancer starts to metastasize. Progression also requires inflammation.

It would appear that extended inflammation almost chronic can aid cancer growth. There are many incidence that show that full blown cancer can develop, if the tissue containing the induced cells is inflamed.

The conclusion is that if new drugs are developed to control inflammation, cancer will be prevented from developing and the individual will live with induced cancer state forever or until something else causes death. Those drugs are in development, but not here at this time.

The inflammatory response as cause of cancer is still in question. Also, it is obvious that many different causes create cancer, and there are many different cancers. It is interesting to note in Microbe volume 6, No.3 page 122, that there are by estimate 10 to the 30 – to 10 to the 32 power of bacteriophages. Bacteriophages are viruses that kill and interact with bacteria. Now it stands to reason, that there may be as many if not more viruses that interact with and kill humans and animal cells or the whole being. Even though there are fewer types of humans and animals than types of bacteria, even if we proportion humans/animals to bacteria, we still will be in the 10 to the 15 power. This is still a bunch of possibilities. In this book we have discussed only the viruses that appear to cause cancer. And we touched on the viruses that are deadly or cause changes in cells without killing or producing cancer. We know these viruses by their affects on the cells. But what about viruses that do not appear to create any effect that we are familiar with, how many of these are there. In many of the attempts to cure cancer by variety of means as we discussed in this chapter the following comes through loud and clear – THERE ARE MANY DISEASES OF CANCER, AND EVERY CANCER TYPE HAS MANY CAUSES.

Gleevec is a drug against a form of leukemia [CML] [30]. It was approved for that use. The drug has been a success, since many patients with this disease have no symptoms of the disease after treatment. But, it appears that some of the cancer cells remain, and under the right conditions are ready to cause cancer. Unfortunately in other cancers, there are very few if any successes.

The surviving cancer cells turn out to be stem cells that have become cancerous. It would appear that stem cells that become cancerous are the beginning of cancer, versus the somatic cell becoming cancerous.

Stem cells are the cells that replace dying and dead cells in the body.

Stem cells are derived from the bone marrow cells called hematopoietic stem cells [HSC]. If the stem cells are to differentiate, the stem cells splits in half and one becomes differentiated while the other cell remains. As the need arises for more stem cells to differentiate, the process continues. One half is preserved until the being dies.

The reason why cancer develops in stem cells is based on the facts that tem cells like cancer cells have many similarities. Cancer cells multiply indefinitely like stem cells. If cancer started in somatic cells, they would be limited in how many times they can divide. Metastasis is similar to stem cells migrating to distal tissues. Stem cells can differentiate into variety of cells in organs and tissues, so does cancer cells. Stem cells are strictly regulated, Remove the regulation and end result is cancer. Also, during differentiation of cancer stem cells, cells result that are not cancerous and everything in between. Radiation and chemotherapy destroys these cells, but not completely, some survive. If the original cancerous cells survive, the cancer redevelops. We do not know at this time, how far during differentiation, if not destroyed, the cells cannot produce cancer. Or maybe, the original stem cell that gave rise to the differentiating stem cell is the culprit. And, the differentiating stem cells cannot form cancer. At this time we just do not know.

It is believed that most if not all cancers are caused by viruses [29]. Viruses that infect the cell and become latent viruses. This can take place many times during an individuals lifetime, or many latent viruses can be inherited, All of these latent viruses are controlled by DNA inhibitor proteins. These viruses do not take over the DNA of the cell to make 300+viruses, rupture the cell and release the viruses. The latent virus, if the right mutation takes place, can take over and run the cell. It cannot escape by making 300+viruses, and therefore uses the cell to do its bidding. Like viruses, it grows by uncontrolled division. It spreads by metastacis like a virus. How are these mutations caused? We are exposed to carcinogens, like tobacco smoke, alcohol, sunshine, grilled meat, cervical papilloma virus, asbestos; but only tiny minority do suffer from cancer.

Gibbs also believe that cancer is a disease of DNA. In 1981 according to Gibbs, that is when the first cancer gene was discovered. Mutations in genes, faulty DNA repair, or errors in DNA copy before division. By 2003, they found 350 genes that most likely can be associated with cancer. This is not in a single cancer, these genes were found in collection of many cancers. What is so surprising is that Collins & Baker in this article proposes to compare the DNA of a cancer cell with the DNA of normal cell. In my opinion, that should have been done 30 years ago. By now we would have a library of differences in the genes of cancer DNA and normal cell DNA for many types of cancer within an organ. I suspect that we will find many differences between the various cancers within a singe organ.

It is also interesting to note that many drugs were developed against surface proteins and other end products of specific genes. For instance, Gleevec, a drug against enzyme, Herceptin against cellular signal receiving protein. Other drugs are again designed to specific single proteins.

In the process of using surgery, radiation, and chemotherapy cures have been accomplished. Many of the survivors for 5 years or more, probably are cancer free because the immune system was activated. It was not because the surgery or radiation or chemotherapy or all three did the job. As it was reviewed in other sections of the Scientific American, and which clearly indicated that the reviewed and presently available cancer treatments attest to this.

Cells have two copies of every chromosome except the X & Y chromosomes. Therefore it takes two hits to knock out both alleles of tumor suppressor gene. There are two copies of the same genes which are called alleles, because there are two sets of chromosomes. 4 – 10 mutations in the right genes can transform any cell. New technologies now allow researchers to survey large fractions of the genomes of cancerous and precancerous cells that have been taken directly from people.

Many recent observations seem to contradict the idea that mutations to a few specific genes lie at the root of all cancers.

Anthony J Luksas PhD

Note: As stated before, cells infected by virus in most cases the virus destroys the cell by releasing 300+ viruses. But, in one in a million the cell is not destroyed but becomes part of the cell's DNA. Under proper conditions, the virus causes the cell to become cancerous that is the next best thing if not able to replicate. Again, since it cannot become a virus and reproduce into 300+ viruses, cancer is the outcome.

In human cancer and in most cancerous cells there are large pieces of chromosomes hooked together and duplications or losses of whole chromosomes. Cancer biologist call such cells aneuploidy. One could assume from virus biology and virus duplication as discussed before, that if a virus cannot reproduce, the virus causes cancer. Note that the chromosomal aberrations are consistent with virus duplication. The virus takes over the cell's DNA, splinters the DNA in forming new viruses. What the above discussed aberations indicate is that the virus in trying to duplicate itself and produce 300+ viruses. In the process of doing so, it splinters the host DNA either completely and produce new viruses, or goes only that far depending on the virus type, and in not being able to reproduce, causes the cell to become cancerous

In this article, Collins and Baker stated that pinpointing the genes involved in cancer will help chart a new course across the complex landscape of human malignancies [9].

In this book Dr. Collins talks about specific genes that were isolated that were different in certain cells, like cancer cells compared to normal cells [8]. The genetic code of humans has been solved. They know essentially all the genes in human cell. As I understand from reading this book, they have developed a method to look at expressed genes versus total genes in the human genome. This is one of the essential steps in my proposal for curing cancer, and will be discussed.

Finally "How to Cure Cancer"

1. NON SELF
   The reason why cancer is cancer, is because the body's immune system does not recognize that the cancer cells have become non self. In order for the body or its immune system to recognize that the cancer cells are non -self, we have to expose components in cancer cell to the immune system. Components that make cancer cell what it is, as opposed to the regular cell that the cancer cell has developed from. To do that, we have to transfer the genes that produce cancer to another organism that will produce these components and cause the body to destroy cancer cells.

   In the past, we were dealing with bacterial infections. How did we destroy many bacterial diseases? We found other bacteria that had enough components similar to the pathogen but not pathogenic to the human.

   Viruses are more integrated into the DNA of the cell, or for that matter other DNA like bacterial DNA. Therefore, we to date have not found genetically changed cells, but not cancerous , that we could use to immunize or cause the body's immune system to recognize and destroy

2. Cells Transformed and not Transformed.
   Cancer cells live forever like the stem cells. Cancer either is a stem cell problem, or the cancer cell has cancelled the genes for apoptasis in somatic cells.

3. Gene Comparison.
   DNA sequencing is being done for many reasons. Forensics uses sequencing and then gel electrophoresis to compare DNA. Bacteriologists

or microbiologists use the DNA sequencing to identify microbes.

If we looked at embryonic cell before differentiation into organs and tissues, we would probably find that most of the DNA was active. During differentiation many areas of the DNA are shut off my methylation. I would suspect, that some of the inactive DNA is viral, acquired through generations or acquired during living.

We may have to go to the stem cells in each organ that is cancerous to find the ground zero DNA for comparison between non- cancerous cell and cancer cell. In any event, we should compare both non- cancerous stem cells from the cancerous organ and non cancerous somatic cells from the cancerous organ and non cancerous somatic cells from that same organ with the cancer cells of the same organ.

4. Genes that are present in Transformed and non Transformed, or expressed only in each case . Transformed and not transformed – determine the genes that are expressed in each case and find the genes that are different in the transformed cells. The difference in expressed and not dormant genes.

5. Note: If you find different genes in transformed and not transformed, including dormant and expressed. This is due to infection of virus in the transformed cells in that individual during his or her lifetime and not inherited. Otherwise, compare total gene compliment against transformed and look at expressed and not expressed. Also note: Besides integrated viruses in the DNA of the individual, inherited or acquired during the individuals life time, there are other DNA in the cell. Bacteria can

integrate the acquired virus into the bacterial DNA [episome] or the virus can be free in the cytoplasm [plasmid]. We should not ignore this fact in human viral DNA. Therefore, look for plasmids in human cytoplasm. Also, mitochondria has bacterial type of DNA – single stranded. Compare the mitochondrial DNA of transformed and not transformed.

Transformation or Genetic changes that are good or bad for the individual are acquiring continuously in microbes and man.

As stated before, there are estimated 10 to the 30th power bacteriophages that can infect bacterial cells only a relatively few have been looked at, because they surfaced as medical or industrial significance, the rest nobody knows. Also, as discussed before, in order for plant gall or nitrogen fixation to take place, the bacteria causing each have to be infected by a specific virus. There are also strong indication that bacteria can transfer DNA to mammals.

6. Amplify.

In order to work with the genes that are expressed in cancer cells, but not found in normal cells somatic or stem cells] the genes have to be multiplied. This process is called AMPLIFICATION. It is done in forensics and in microbial identification.

7. Put genes from transformed [different] into non -pathogenic non toxin producing B. subtilis. It is one of the most studied microbes, used to produce many chemicals, and it's genetic map is known. Microbe,4/2011, p.176 Bio Cyc: microbial genomes and cellular networks. Make sure that the bacteria chosen is killed by a normal antibiotic, i.e., with and without the cancer genes. The bacteria may

also be attenuated by adjuvant like most antigens today.

8. Destroy the supressors in this bacteria, make these genes to be expressed without feedback inhibition.

9. Prepare the bacteria as antigen, or inject these bacteria into the cancer patient.

10. The human immunity will recognize these as non self and start destroying the bacteria as well as the cancer.

There are very rare cases were a antibody has been produced in the body of the cancer patient that kept the cancer in check, and not destroyed the cancer. In these cases the antibody may start destroying some organ or organs. Only after the cancer is removed by surgery and the antibody level decreases that the individual can live if the cancer has been removed early enough so that only insignificant damage has been done.

This phenomenon may take place in this approach to cancer. But, I suspect that this will not be the case since in the above case it takes a long time for the destruction of organs to take place. This approach to cancer should be swift in curing cancer. Once the cancer cells are destroyed the antibodies to the cancer gene products will decrease but not like in the above case.

11. FDA will have a problem with this approach, therefore, test with animal models. By the way, FDA would not have allowed Pasture to do the injections like against rabies, and others, or TB using the cow TB organism.

The trick is to cause the body to identify the cancer cells and destroy the cancer cells. Cancer cells form throughout our lifetime, but the body immune system identifies it as non -self and destroys the cancer cell or cells before it forms a colony.

Today chemotherapy and radiation that is used destroys growing cells like immune system as well as cancer cells. Therefore immunity is suppressed if not eliminated. No chemotherapy or radiation destroys all cancer cells, the process only prolongs life. Unless the suppressed immune system recognizes the cancer cells as non self, and in spite of it's suppression starts to attack the cancer.

Today and in the past, we are looking for the magic bullet for cancer like Erlich did for bacterial infections. He did not find it, I suspect nor are we going to find one against cancer. Since there are so many potential genes that are active in cancer. And the same type of cancer may have different genes causing it. Note that not unlike in bacteria were there is a possibility of 10 to the 30th types of bacteriophages, in humans there may be less, since there are many more bacteria types then human species. There may be as many as 10 to the 10th power. We only are aware of the viruses that manifest themselves in humans, what about the rest of 10 to the 10th. What are these doing in humans? If one is looking for a magic bullet, which most research in cancer are doing, it is like looking for a needle in a hay stack. Sometime drugs against these "needles in a hay stack" do bear fruit. But, there is no drug to date that cures every cancer patient completely, some survive 5 years, in few the cancer is not detected. I believe, the few where cancer disappeared , can be explained by the treatment somehow caused the immune system to recognize the cancer cells as non self, and destroy the cancer. The only solution to cancer is to do what is recommended.

In the old days bacteria as to genus, species, subspecies, and strains were identified by their fermentation patterns. Does the bacteria utilize certain sugars, amino acids, grow on certain media to mention a few. The book, Bergey's Manual of Determinative Bacteriology, describes the various media used to identify a particular bacteria. Today, they use genetic typing. They extract the DNA, splinter it into genes. Next they run gel electrophoreses, and compare the patterns of genes in the gel.

The process is relatively simple today, it was not in the beginning.

The cancer cure approach presented as a theory, looks complicated – and it is. But, the components are already in place, all we have to do is apply the procedures. And in time, machines will be set up to produce antigens from cancer genes for injection into cancer patients.

This cancer treatment approach started in 1957, when I took my first course in microbiology. It took all these years to finalize how to do it. During the years the various components were developed to fit into the concept. Like the book "The language of God" clearly showed that these are procedures to identify expressed and not expressed genes. There were other key developments that were developed during the incubation time.

I sincerely hope, that research into cancer cause changes course, and starts developing results that cure cancer completely. Lets stop looking for the needle in the hay stack or Erlich's magic bullet, lets start serious research.

By the way, during treatment with the proposed procedure, the cancer patient will have to be kept alive, especially the terminal cases. To do this, we may put the patient on Vitamin C treatment, or in some cases on chemotherapy, but eventually as the above treatment takes hold, cancer should disappear.

It also is important to note, that there may be more than one cancer in an individual at one time, or developed during various treatments that individual has gone through. Need to check not only the primary tumor but also secondary or, so- called, metastasized tumors for genes. If different genes are found, that is a different cancer. The new cancer has to be treated separately by the above procedure.

Also, this procedure should be considered for preventing cancer. We have determined in some cases, if a particular gene is present that person has a better than average chance of developing the cancer associated with that gene. The presence of a specific gene in women makes them more susceptible to cancer of the breast. It is to be noted, that cancers of the breast develop in women without that particular gene. Breast cancer therefore is a group of diseases. In many cases the women chooses to have her breasts removed to prevent cancer, especially if this type of cancer runs in the family. This is an extreme procedure that in my opinion should be replaced by the above immunization procedure, after the procedure has been proven to work.

In the cervical cancer, there are also genes indicating the increase potential in cervical cancer. That gene or genes have been identified and these genes are found in a specific virus. People with these specific genes that also are found in specific viruses, can be immunized against that virus. As cancer genes are identified with specific virus, that virus should be used to immunize, not unlike in cervical cancer. But, do not use viruses as vehicles for cancer genes, if these genes were not found in that particular virus – THIS IS A POTENTIAL FOR CREATING NEW AND EVEN MORE DANGEROUS VIRUSES. It seems to prevent cervical cancers but not all. It is probably that cervical cancer is a group of cancers not just one. As times goes on more genes will be found to be associated with specific cancers. These genes should be incorporated into the above immunization scheme to prevent that particular cancer.

If the genes identified can be without doubt associated with a specific virus, use the virus to immunize. I suspect, in many cases there will not be a clear association with a specific virus, in those cases use the procedure described in this book, again once it is proven. It should not be hard to prove, since cervical cancer immunization is done with a virus. In the proposed procedure, if a virus containing the cancer genes cannot be found, again do not use a virus to immunize after the cancer genes have been incorporated in that virus. Use the suggested bacteria to incorporate the cancer genes into for immunization. The possibility of bacteria transferring genes is a remote possibility in this situation.

Chapter 8 References.

1. AARP, May 2008, Good News About Cancer.
2. Gina Barikata, Cell Surface Protein: No Simple Cancer Mechanisms, science, Vol. 190, Oct. 3, 1975, p.39.
3. Abbas M. Benbebani, The Small Pox Story: Historical Perspective, ASM News, Vol. 57, No.11, 1991.
4. Erwin Cameron and Linus Pauling, The Orthomolecular Treatment of Cancer I, The Role of Ascorbic Acid in Host Resistance, Chem. Biol. Interactions, 9, 1974, p. 273.
5. Erwin Cameron and Allan Campbell, The Orthomolecular Treatment of Cancer II, Chem. Biol. Interactions, 9, 1974, P. 285.
6. Erwin Cameron and Linus Pauling, Supplimental Ascorbate in the Supportive Treatment of Cancer: Prolongation of Survival Time in Terminal Human Cancer, Proc. Natl. Sci. USA, Vol. 78, No. 10, p. 3685.

7. Stanley H. Cohen, et al., Construction of Biologically Functional Bacterial plasmids in Vitro, Proc. Nat. Acad. Sci., USA, Vol. 70, No. 11, Nov. 1973, p.3240.
8. Francis S. Collins, The language of God, Free Press, 2006.
9. Francis S. Collins and Anna B. Baker, Mapping the Cancer Genome, Scientific American, Sept. 30, 2008, p.22.
10. Could a DNA Test Help You ? Orlando Sentinel, Sept. 21, 2008.
11. P. J. Fishinger, et al., Reversion of Murine Sarcoma Virus Transformed Mouse Cells: Variance Without a Sarcoma Virus, Science, Vol. 176, June 2, 1972.
12. Emil Frei III, The National Cancer Chemotherapy Program, Science, Vol. 217, Aug. 13, 1982, p.600.
13. Peter Gwynne, Gene Therapy Enters Era of Ambiguous Promise, R.D. Magazine, Oct. 1995.
14. S. Harguinbey and R. C. Kolbeck Cancer – A Generalization, American Laboratory, 1976, p.71.
15. S. Harguinbey and M. Gillis, Experimental and Human Cancer, pH and Spontaneous Regressions, American Laboratory, Aug. 1976, p. 91.
16. Jean L. Marx, Tumor Immunology [I]: The Host Response to Cancer, Science, Vol. 184, Issue 4136, May. 3, 1974, p.552.
17. Jean L. Marx, Tumor Immunology [II]:Strategies for Cancer Therapy, Science, Vol. 184, issue 4136, May 3, 1974.
18. Thomas H. Maugh II, Chemotherapy: Antiviral Agents Come Of Age, Science, Vol. 192, 1982, p. 128.
19. Dennis J. McCance, Human Tumor Viruses, Published by ASM Press, 1998.
20. Linda Milo Ohr, A Growing Arsenal Against Cancer, Food Technology, Vol. 56, No. 7, July, 2002, p.67.

21. Angela M. Miraglio and R. D. Feeding, The Fight Against Cancer, food product Design, Aug. 2003, p. 29.
22. No Name, Bacterial Vectors for Delivering Gene and Anticancer Therapies, ASM News, Microbe, March 2011, p. 115.
23. No Name, How are they Different from Normal Cells and Why do they Escape Immune Destruction, Laboratory Management, July 1973, p. 38.
24. No Name, Spontaneous Regression of Cancer: Hope and Warnings, laboratory management, July 1974, p.16.
25. Eugene W. Nester, at al., Microbiology, Molecules, Microbes and Man, 1973, Holt Rinehart and Winston, Inc.
26. Garth L. Nicolson, Cancer Metastasis, mature, Aug. 1976, p. 66.
27. Justin O. Neway, Fermentation process Development of Industrial Organisms, 1989, Publisher Marcel Dekker, Inc.
28. Martin C. Raff, Cell Surface Immunology, Scientific American, 234: 30 – 39, 57.
29. W. Wayt Gibbs, Understanding the Root of Cancer, Scientific American, Sept. 2008, p. 31.
30. Michael F. Clarke and Michael W. Becker, Stem Cells: The Real Culprid in Cancer, scientific American, Sept. 2008, p. 40.
31. Gerry Stix, a Malignant Flame, Scientific American, Sept. 2008, p.48.
32. Jacques Banchereau, The Long Arm of the Immune Sustem, Sept. 2008.
33. Rakesh K. Jain, Taming Vessels to Treat Cancer, Scientific American, Sept. 2008, p. 64.

34. Dirk M. Nettelbeck, Ronald D. Alvarez and David T. Curiel, Tumor – Busting Viruse, Scientific American, Sept. 2008, p. 72.
35. Francisco J. Esteva and Gabriel N. Hortobagyi, Gaining Ground on Breast Cancer, Scientific American, Sept. 2008,p.88.
36. Hyun S. Shin, et al., Immunotherapy of Cancer with Antibody, Science, Vol. 194, Oct. 15, 1976, p. 327.
37. Current Topics, Cellular Apoptosis: On Death and Dying, ASM News, Vol. 60, No12, 1994.
38. Scientific American, p.80, Nick Lane, New Light on Medicine, Use of Light to Cure Cancer.